SOMATIC EXERCISES

FOR
BEGINNERS

KRISTEN PAYTON

TABLE OF CONTENTS

INTRODUCTION

- ACKNOWLEDGEMENTS
- BOOK'S STRUCTURE
- THEORETICAL INTRODUCTION
- CONSISTENCY IS THE SECRET
- HOW TO STAY MOTIVATED

EXERCISES

HOW TO DOWNLOAD YOUR BONUSES

SCAN THE QR CODE:

INTRODUCTION

ACKNOWLEDGEMENTS

I thank you sincerely for purchasing this book on somatic exercises. I am so happy that you chose to start this amazing discipline that is changing so many lives around the world. You have just taken the first steps towards a healthier and better life! These kinds of exercises will allow you to create a straight connection between your body and mind, improving the physical awareness in a noticeably brief time. There are thousands of people who practice this discipline every single day and who are having impressive results! Are you ready to start this adventure with me?

BOOK'S STRUCTURE

The book is made in a quite simple and friendly way; indeed, each exercise will accept two pages of it. On the left page, I have included all the textual details you need to perform in maximum safety. On the right one, you will find photos that will help you understand exactly the movements you will have to conduct. However, I have chosen to give you free access to all the explanatory videos. I suggest you to always watch them to be sure you encompass the exercise without risking unnecessary injuries. Finally, I created a workout routine that you will be able to find at the end of this manual. I thought a lot before writing it down. However, I decided to create amazingly simple and friendly charts that can be consulted comfortably during training. Each table contains the list of exercises you will have to perform on that day. I hope everything is clear and that you are satisfied with your purchase. Finally, I want to advise you to use a personal diary to track all your progress over time. Do not hesitate to take a few minutes at the end of each workout to record the sensations you felt during your workout and the future goals you set for your wellness. Now you have all the resources you need to start this amazing journey! I really wish you the best!

THEORETICAL INTRODUCTION

I know that, during your life, you will have tried several ways to get fit, but you have never tried somatic exercises. Indeed, this discipline is little-known, but it is spreading very quickly, thanks to social media. Many people have started practicing it, desiring to keep the right shape to find a sense of balance and interior harmony.

CONSISTENCY IS THE SECRET

Unfortunately, every day I see people who give up after 1 or 2 weeks, losing motivation. This is the main reason people are frustrated and stressed out. You already know that training with consistency is fundamental, especially if you desire to achieve hugely noteworthy results and I am not just talking about physical results (weight loss, toning, etc.), but also, from a mental point of view. This discipline is one of the few that can create a connection between body and mind. This book will help you keep your shape by preventing several diseases and improving the quality of your life by promoting mental wellness, which is very underestimated, but extremely important. Do not forget that regular workout stimulates the endorphins production which can reduce stress and anxiety. All these elements will lead to an especially important improvement in your mood and an increase in productivity as your body will be stronger and your mind will be increasingly more relaxed. Remember that training is nothing more than an act of care and love towards ourselves!

HOW TO STAY MOTIVATED

Unfortunately, I have met few motivated people. Indeed, most of them, who start any physical activity, give up after a few weeks. The causes are different, but we can attribute them to the absence of objectives and purposes. That is why I wanted to include this essential paragraph in which I will give you some practical suggestions on how to stay motivated when you feel tired or unprofitable.

SET CLEAR GOALS

Before starting the 30-day program, I recommend you take 30-40 minutes to reflect on your purposes and write them down in a large notebook! You do not have to create a long text, simple, clear, and direct bullet points are enough. Writing suggestions to concretize thoughts and make more practicable goals. This is an approach based on clarity and specificity that can be effective eventually. Doing that provides direction and makes it easier to track progress and celebrate successes. Do you know what is meant by "clear goals"? Do not be worried! I will explain it to you! There must be a clear purpose.

- specific
- measurable
- reachable
- realistic

It makes no sense to set yourself elusive goals like "I want to improve my flexibility." This is not a measurable purpose, because it is too generic; in fact, it would be impossible to measure progress. An example of a clear goal: "I want to increase my legs' flexibility and be able to touch my toes with my hands within three months from now." Remember that only these kinds of objectives can be controlled over time. Therefore, I invite you to set yourself the most specific ones possible so that you know exactly what you want to achieve and how you need to do to get there. Choose achievable and realistic goals by considering your initial situation. It is useless to hope to reach significant physical results in a noticeably short week because our body needs time to change, being adapted to your new rhythms. People who hope to lose weight in a noticeably brief time, do not lose a single kilo, turning into very frustrated subjects!

WHAT IS THE BEST WAY TO SET CLEAR GOALS?

The best feasible way to think about clear goals is to follow a structured process. Firstly, I suggest you do an inner reflection, asking yourself what you hope to achieve from somatic exercises and how your life could improve. This type of practice is called introspection and can help you meditate on your body and mind. Once you have identified your purposes, you will need to break them down into smaller ones. Each of them can have different deadlines. That is why I recommend using a diary to keep track of everything, otherwise you risk forgetting. You will realize that progress will be gradual but regular, reaching small intermediate goals will support you to keep your motivation extremely high. When you annotate them, remember to also include a specific deadline, by creating a sense of urgency and planning the actions you must perform to achieve everything by that date you set previously. Try to review them periodically to reach your progress and make changes, if you think it is necessary. It is essential to be flexible, adapting your objectives as you get better with your workout, as unexpected events may emerge.

SET THE REWARDS

Besides the purpose definition, I advise you to establish rewards once you reach it. The most important thing is that they are so meaningful, helping you stay motivated even in the most complicated circumstances. I will give you some ideas to implement in your life:

- a relaxing day in the swimming pool
- a wellness treatment
- a dinner with your own friends your favorite food

These are just a few examples. You try to identify the best rewards for you.

SHARE YOUR GOALS WITH OTHER PEOPLE

I guarantee you that this is a very impressive activity because I have personally used it for an exceedingly long time in sport and professional life. I suggest you try it because it is motivating as it creates a sense of responsibility and effort that can encourage you to always give your best during the workout. I usually share my purposes with my friends or relatives, and it helps me very much.

CREATE YOUR ROUTINE

Everyone has different individual and professional commitments that often occupy most of the day. The only way to be sure of achieving your purposes is to plan yourself as best as you can, choosing specific times and places to do your exercises. Creating a routine is fundamental for your success. Over the weeks, I managed to make training a consolidated daily habit and I only succeeded thanks to consistency and efforts.

SET A DEFINED HOURS TO DO YOUR WORKOUT

The first step to create a useful routine is to establish a defined time to carry out your own exercises. Selecting a specific moment is helpful to create your new habit, by minimizing the risk of procrastination. I know many people who prefer to train early in the morning or in the evening. It is up to you. Each of us is different and unique and, that is why, it is fundamental to think about your daily commitments in an incredibly careful way.

CHOOSE THE PERFECT SPOT

The benefits of somatic exercises are that you can do your workout easily from home without having to go to the gym every time, wasting a lot of time in the car. Find a room large enough to conduct, erasing all distractions. I do not suggest you train yourself with the television, because you could get distracted and lose concentration. Choose a quiet environment and focus only on training. If you desire to create a more greeting atmosphere you can organize the room with elements that inspire calm and wellness like plants, scented candles, and paintings.

LISTEN TO YOUR BODY

To perform somatic exercises in a remarkably successful and effective way, you need to know how to listen carefully, analysing all the physical, emotional, and mental feelings that each of us experiences during the workout. This approach will allow you to prevent injuries and overloads, but also to understand what your body really needs. Obviously, it takes time to develop this skill. However, I assure you that it can completely change the way you see training. Indeed, you will learn to observe how your body responds to this kind of stimuli. Every movement must be conducted very carefully, trying not to ignore even the smallest pain signals that the body sends us. Pain is a clear indicator that something is wrong. The exercise you are doing is too intense or your execution is incorrect. Do not ignore these sensations and change your training immediately, if necessary. You can choose to adapt the exercises to your needs by changing the training intensity or lengthening the recovery moments. If you feel particularly tired, perform relaxation and deep breathing exercises which can eliminate all the tension accumulated during the day.

IDENTIFY YOUR LIMITS

Remember that physical development is gradual but constant. So, do not push yourself too hard. Do not try to exceed your limits. Listen to your own body and be patient especially during the first workouts. If you have never practiced somatic exercises, do not expect to be able to perform all the movements without difficulty because this may not be the case and it is perfectly normal! Recognize and identify your own limits and do not stop at the first difficulties. Re-read your goals written in your diary and enjoy every single moment during your workouts.

BE PROUD OF YOUR SUCCESS

One of the most effective and useful ways to always have high motivations is to recognize and celebrate your own progress. However, to do this, you need to be constant. Do not forget to use the diary to annotate all the feelings during this amazing path to appreciate this physical and mental transformation. Over time, you will experience emotional, mental, and physical changes that will have a straight impact on your motivation. To track your progress is to take photos of yourself before and after your training program. Subsequently, you should compare them, noticing the physical results you achieve. From a mental point of view, you will feel grateful for having never given up even if you felt frustrated or stressed out. Once you do it, you will cherish the workout and effort you put into this journey. Never give up and keep training until you achieve all your goals.

SHARE YOUR GOALS WITH OTHER PEOPLE

Remember to always involve those you love you and, every time you reach a goal, write it down in your diary. You can choose who to share your successes with, by celebrating even the smallest ones to increase your sense of responsibility and personal satisfaction.

USE CUSTOMIZED POSITIVE DECLARATIONS

Before each exercise, write positive declarations right in your diary. This is particularly effective, especially when motivation is low, because these sentences influence your mind and body in a positive way. Your mental status will change, and you will immediately feel more energetic! Words have an extraordinarily strong power, and they can improve your own mental approach by making you optimistic. I also suggest you erase all negative and self-limiting thoughts, because they do not contribute to your path. Always try to have a positive outlook characterized by a constructive mental attitude that supports you best overcome the obstacles and challenges you will encounter in your existence. This type of positive mental approach should be adopted not only in sport, but also in everyday life as it will help you better face the difficulties. Social media and the internet are full of motivational sentences, but I advise you to personally write customized positive affirmations as they are much more beneficial. Reflect on your goals and desires just to create original declarations and repeat them aloud even during the exercises. Your motivation will allow you to reach the stars!

PARTICIPATE IN GROUP TRAININGS

One of the methods I personally use to train even when I do not want to, is to enjoy group training sessions at my local gym. Doing this, I feel almost "forced" to work on my physical and mental connection, because I am not alone. The most important advantage of this kind of activity is that you can support each other as everyone has the same purpose, which is to improve physically but also mentally.

EXERCISES

1 – STANDING ROCKING

BENEFITS:

- mind-body connection improvement
- back relaxation

HOW TO PERFORM THE EXERCISE

1 Stand in the center of the mat

2 Close the eyes, placing the right hand on your chest and the left one on the abdomen

3 Start swinging to the left and then, to the other side

4 Find your perfect spot and follow the instructions present in the program

TIPS FOR THE MOVEMENT

Always keep your abdomen well-contracted with your legs tense in order not to lose balance. Focus on your pelvis movement and remember to listen always to your body.

BREATHING INDICATIONS

Keep a steady and controlled breathing.

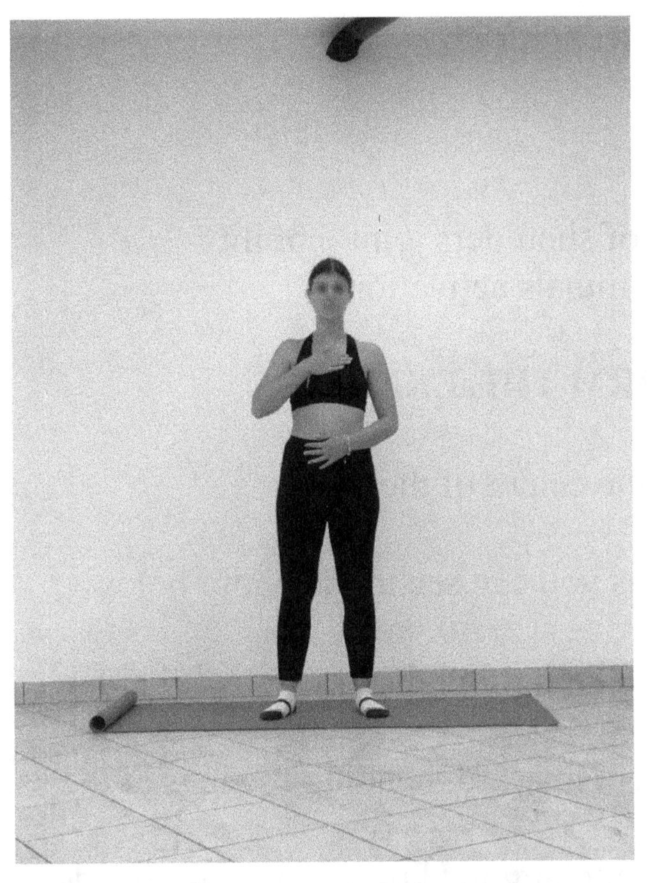

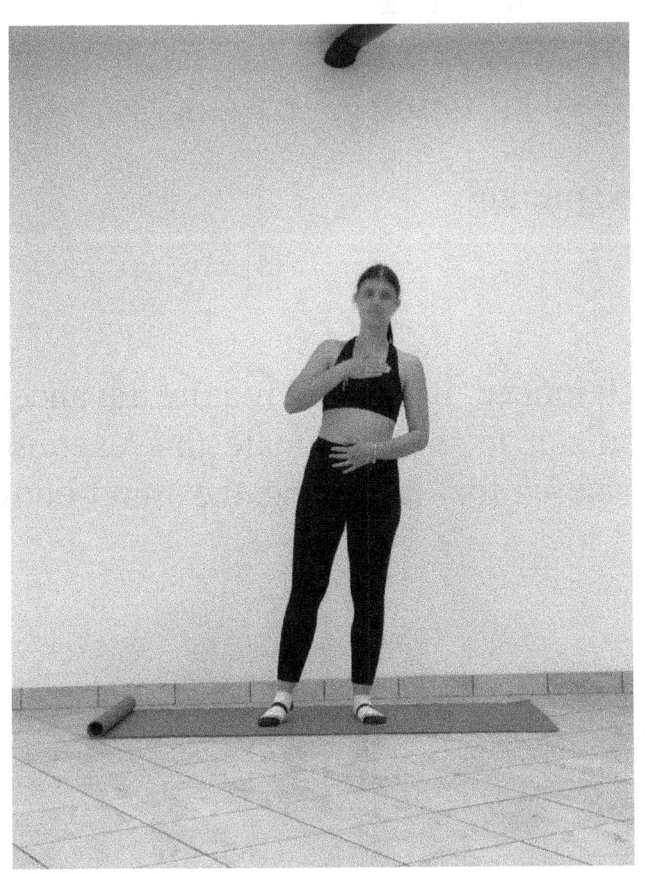

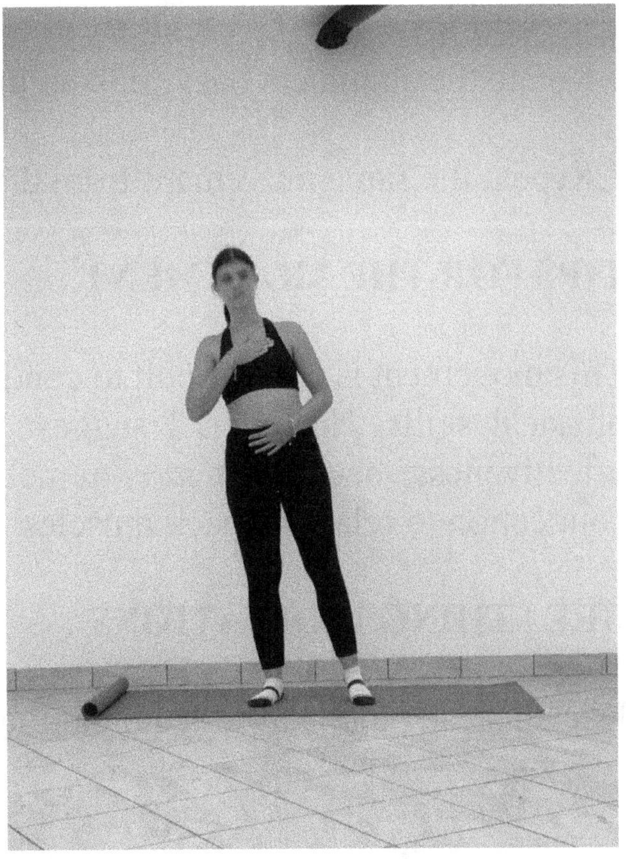

2 – SHOULDERS ROTATION

BENEFITS:

- improvement of shoulders joint mobility
- traps and abdominals activation

HOW TO PERFORM THE EXERCISE

1 Place yourself at the center of the mat

2 Spread your legs as you can see in the photo below

3 Keep the legs straight, putting the arms at your sides

4 Rotate the shoulders forward, bending the legs at the same time

5 Stretch the arms, touching the knees with your hands

6 Rotate the shoulders back, raising the head upwards

7 Repeat the same movement from the beginning

TIPS FOR THE MOVEMENT

This movement is not difficult to conduct; indeed, it does not require advanced physical skills. However, I suggest you not to underestimate this exercise effectiveness, because it is extremely useful for improving the mind-body connection to relax the back muscles.

BREATHING INDICATIONS

Keep a steady and controlled breathing.

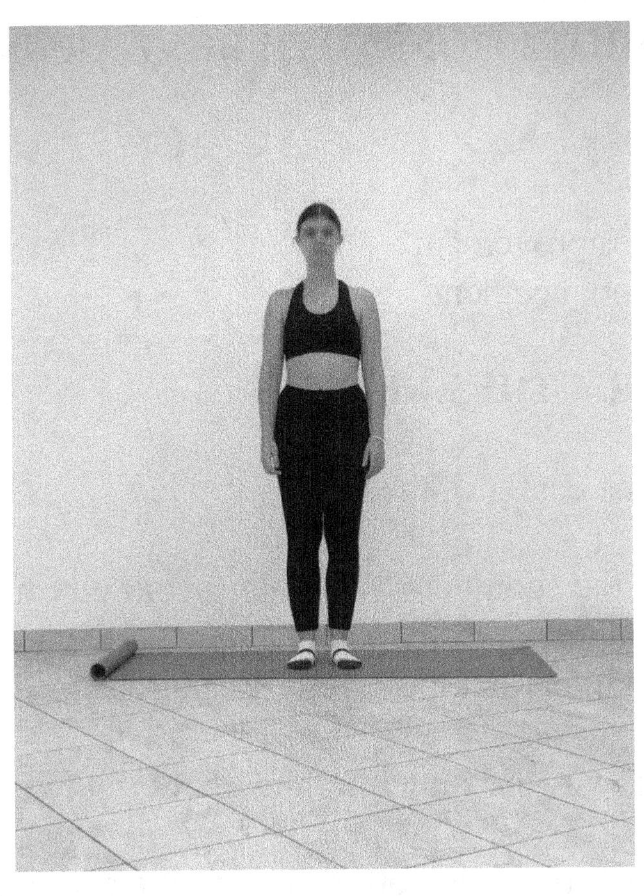

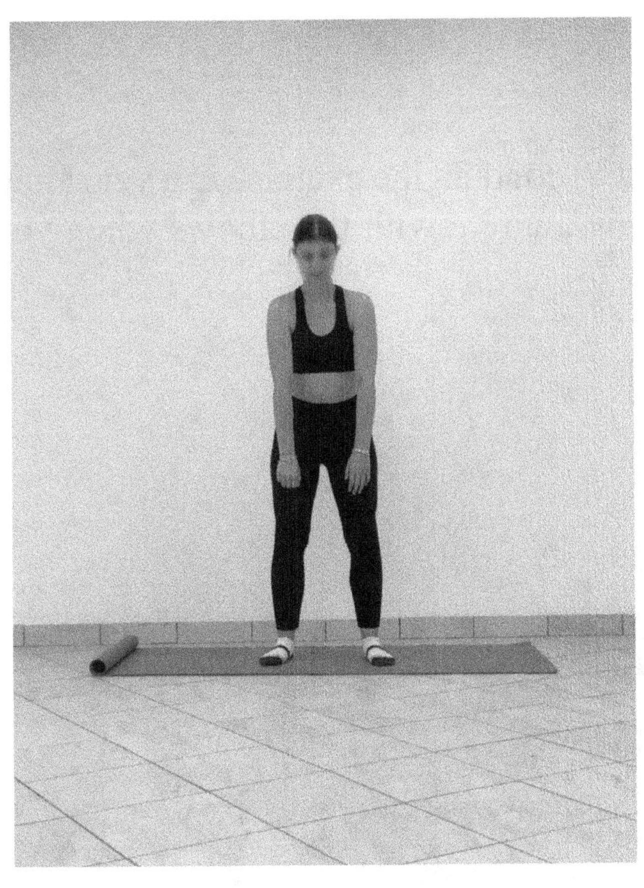

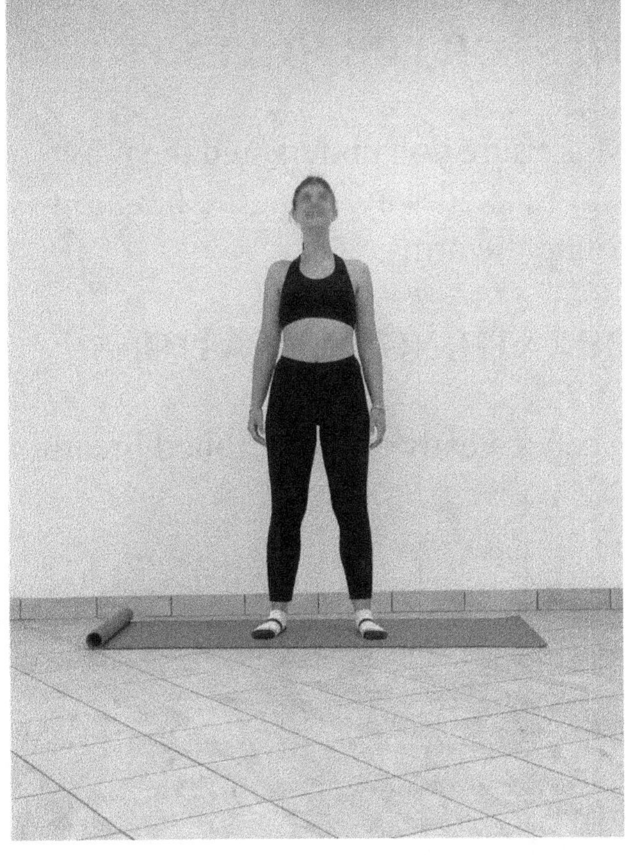

3 – SHOULDERS ROTATIONS WITH BENT ARMS

BENEFITS:

- joint mobility improvement
- coordination enhancement

HOW TO PERFORM THE EXERCISE

1 Place yourself at the center of the mat

2 Put your hands on the shoulders by bending your elbows

3 Rotate the arms counterclockwise forming a circle

4 Stretch the arms downward, touching the knees with your hands

5 Come back to the starting position, repeating the exercise

TIPS FOR THE MOVEMENT

Make sure you understand the movement to conduct the exercise in a very fluid and relaxed way. Imagine having to draw a circle with the elbows when you rotate the arms.

BREATHING INDICATIONS

Keep a steady and controlled breathing.

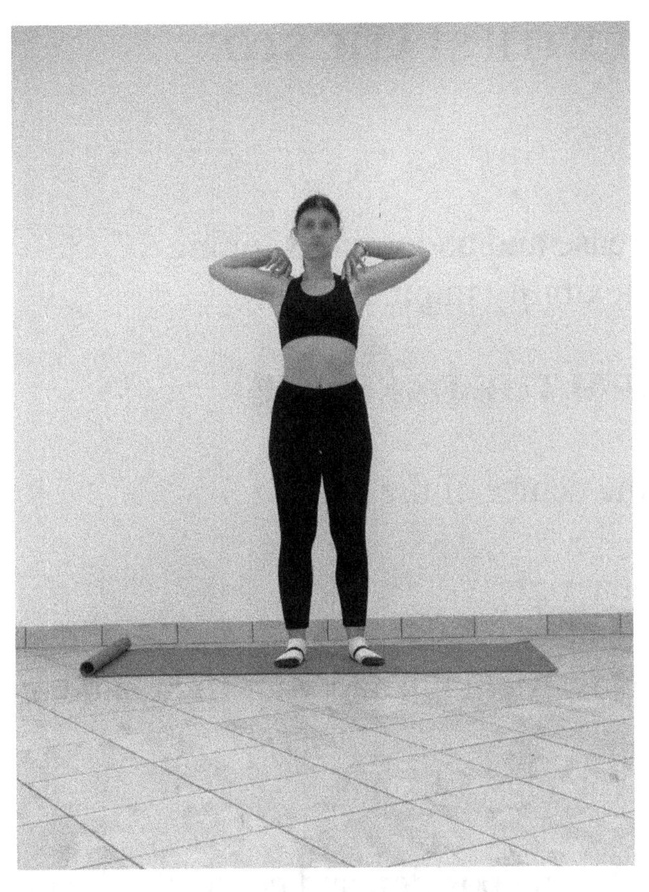

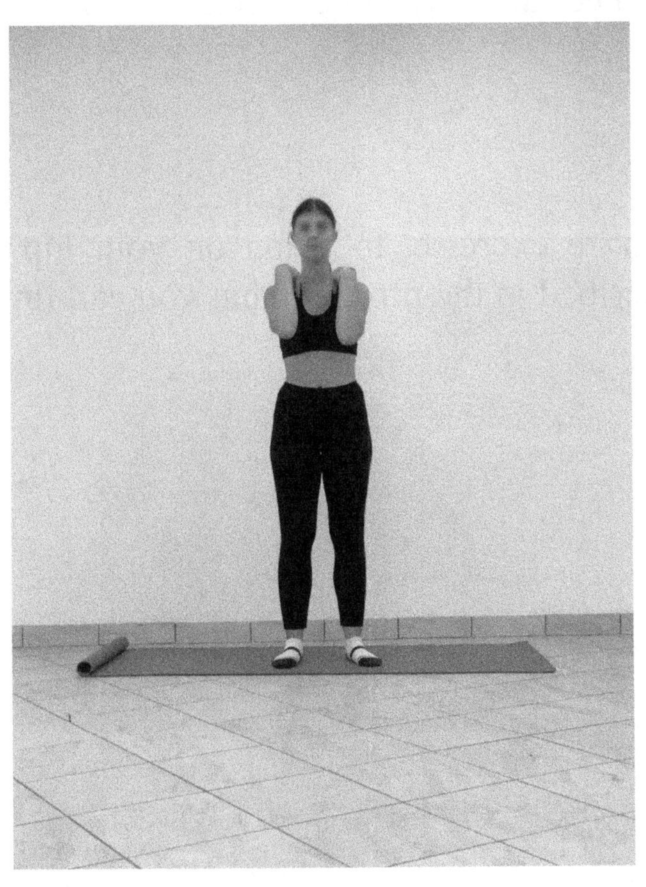

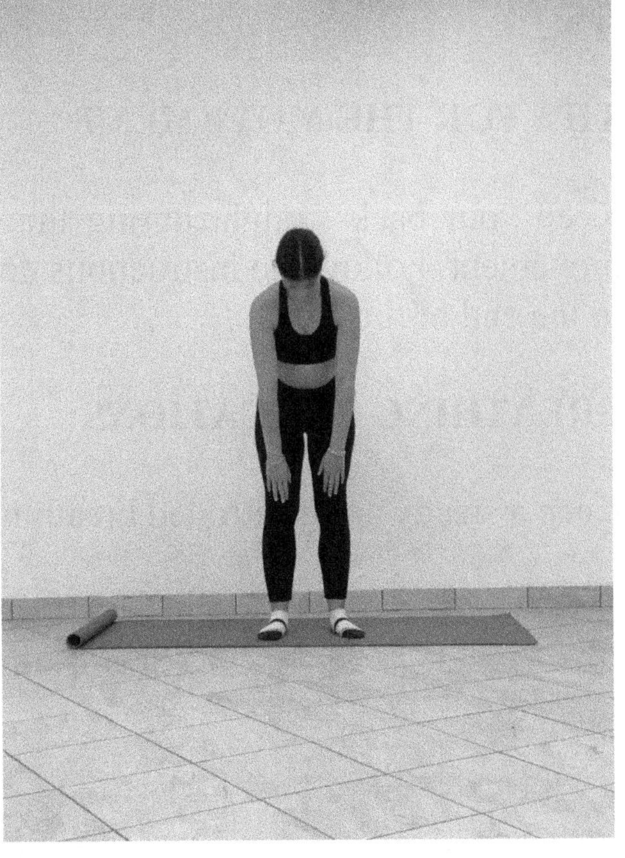

4 – TORSO TWIST WITH STATIC STOP

BENEFITS:

- waist size decrease and abdominals toning
- mobility and flexibility improvement

HOW TO PERFORM THE EXERCISE

1 Place yourself at the center of the mat

2 Twist the torso to the right

3 Put the left hand on the right hip and your right hand on the left gluteus

4 Keep this position for a few seconds

5 Come back to the starting position and conduct the same exercise to the left side

TIPS FOR THE MOVEMENT

Keep your back straight during the entire exercise, focusing on your hip's movement. Follow the instructions described in the program that you can find in the end of this book.

BREATHING INDICATIONS

Keep a steady and controlled breathing.

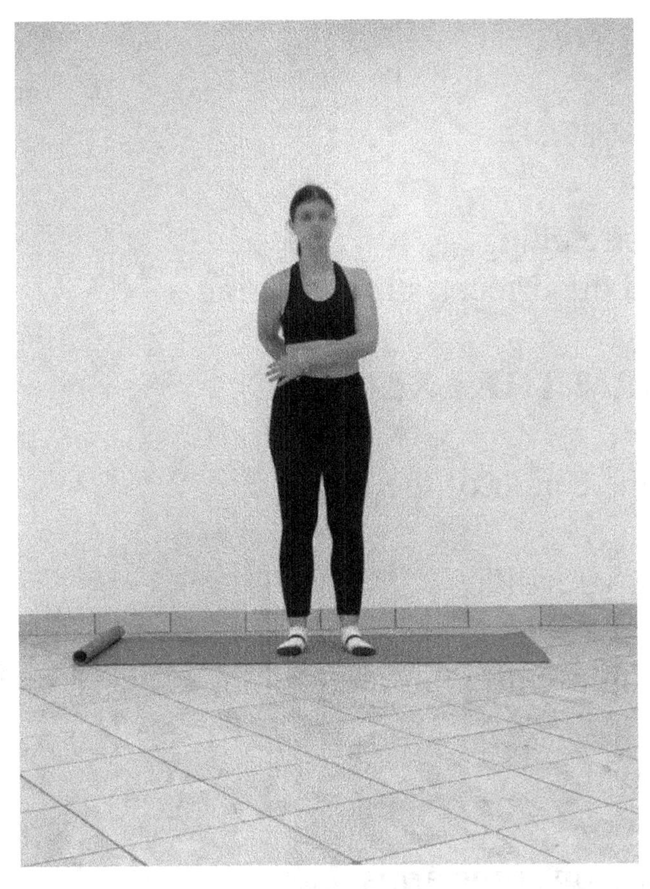

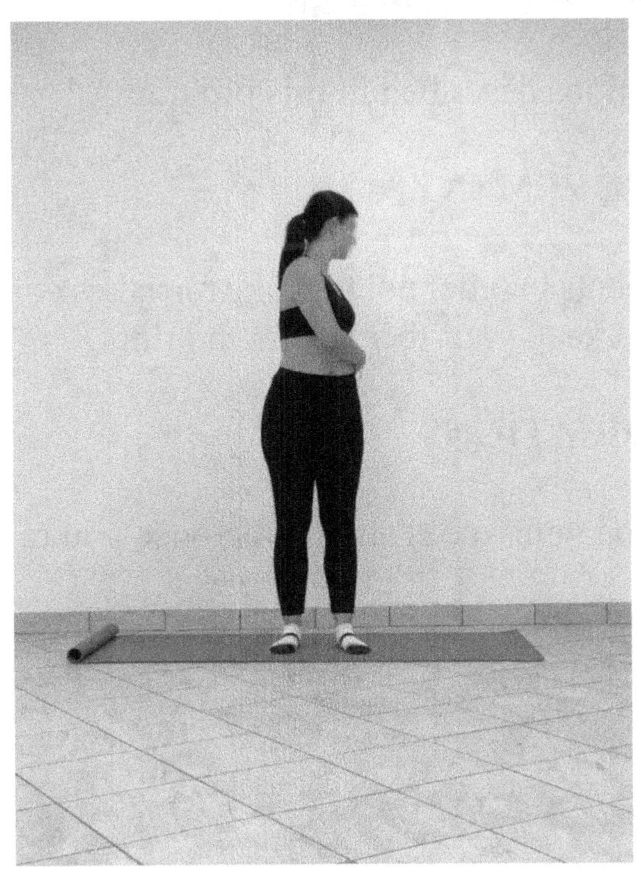

5 – TORSO BENDING

BENEFITS:

- back muscles stretching
- hamstrings and quadriceps strengthening

HOW TO PERFORM THE EXERCISE

1 Place yourself at the center of the mat

2 Extend the arms at your sides

3 Keep the back straight with your abdominal muscles well-contracted

4 Raise the arms upwards

5 Bend the knees and lower the arms

6 Follow the instructions described in this program

TIPS FOR THE MOVEMENT

Learn all the movements in order not to make mistakes during the performance. Spread your legs and keep your feet flat on the floor.

BREATHING INDICATIONS

Exhale once you bend your knees and inhale once you raise your arms.

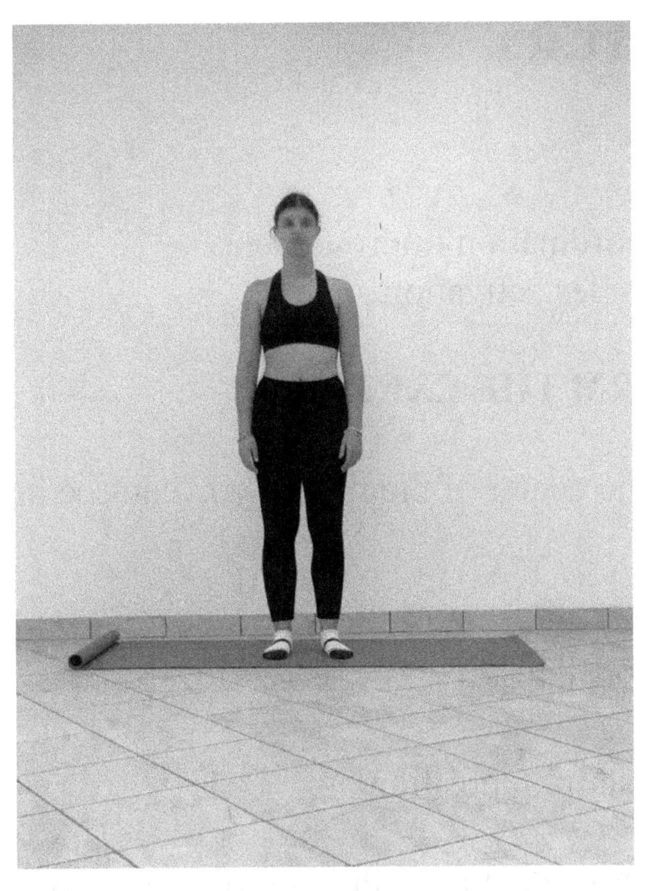

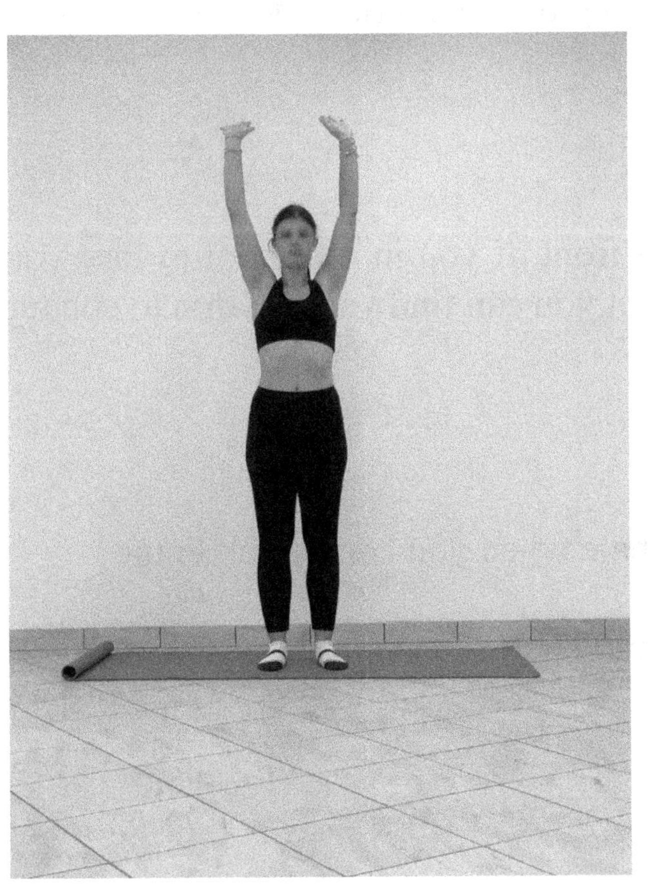

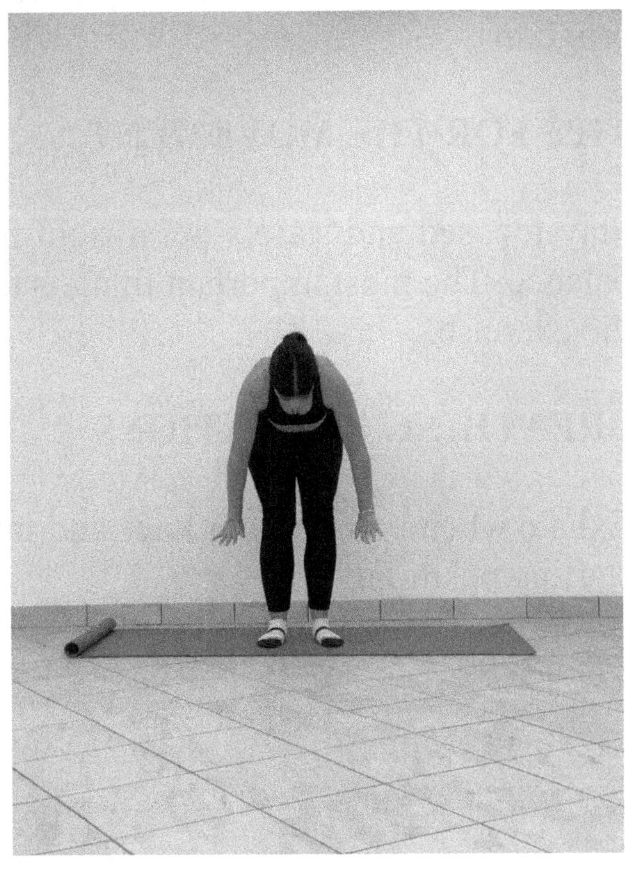

6 – WALKING IN PLACE

BENEFITS:

- balance and coordination improvement
- stabilizing muscles activation

HOW TO PERFORM THE EXERCISE

1 Place yourself at the center of the mat as you can see in the photo below

2 Raise the left knee

3 Put the right hand on the knee

4 Come back to the starting position

5 Repeat the same movement by following the instructions described in the program

TIPS FOR THE MOVEMENT

Stay focused and stare a point right in front of you in order not to lose your balance. The most important thing is that you can find your rhythm to conduct the exercise.

BREATHING INDICATIONS

Exhale when you lift your knee and inhale when you come back to the starting position.

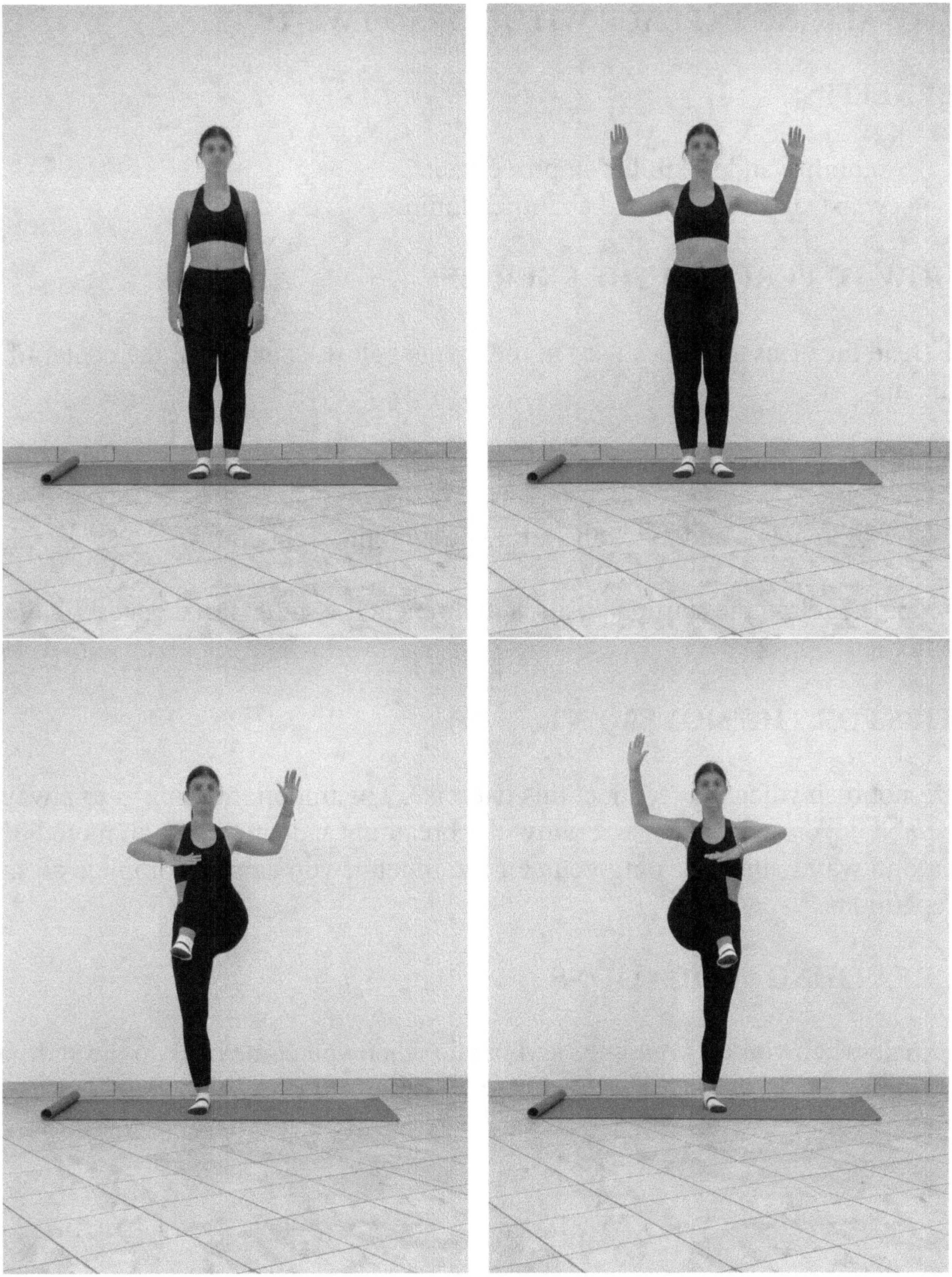

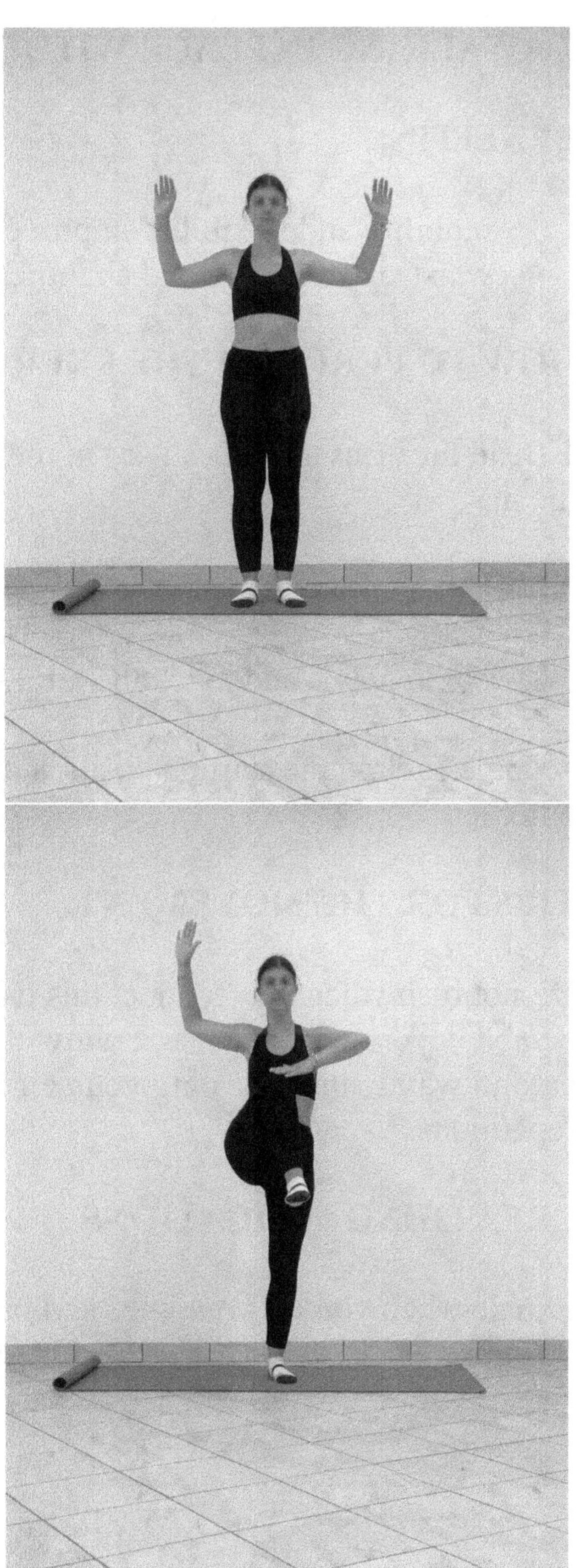

7 – WALKING IN PLACE WITH TORSO TWIST

BENEFITS:

- mobility and flexibility improvement
- waist size decrease and abdomen toning

HOW TO PERFORM THE EXERCISE

1 Bend the arms as you can see in the image below, standing at the center of the mat

2 Raise the left knee

3 Twist the pelvis and touch the left knee with the right elbow

4 Come back to the starting position and repeat the same movement with the other leg

TIPS FOR THE MOVEMENT

Do not rush when you conduct this exercise. The important thing is to always be able to keep the balance. Follow the breathing indications in an incredibly careful way without beating yourself too much if you cannot complete all the repetitions.

BREATHING INDICATIONS

Exhale when you lift your knee and inhale when you come back to the starting position.

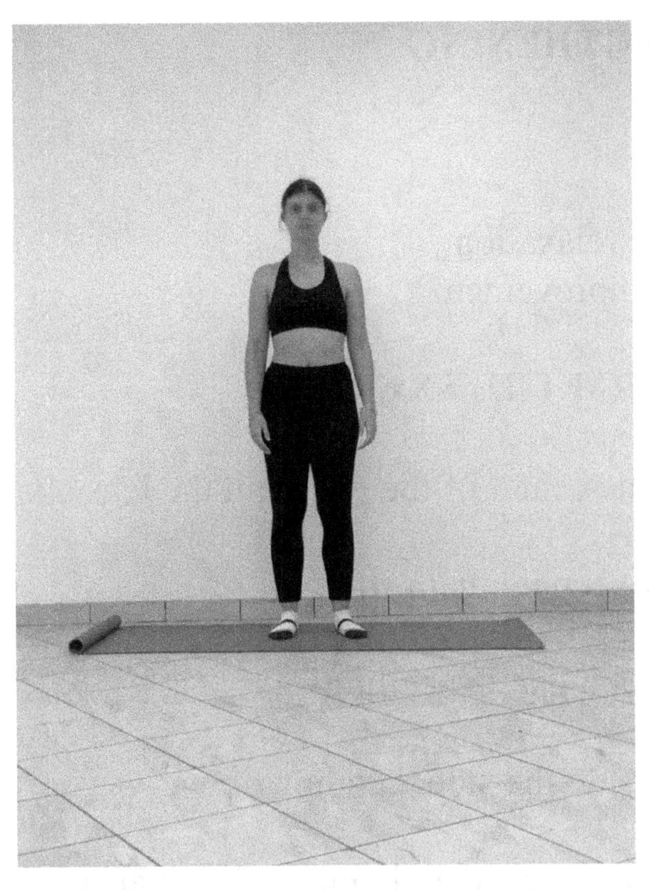

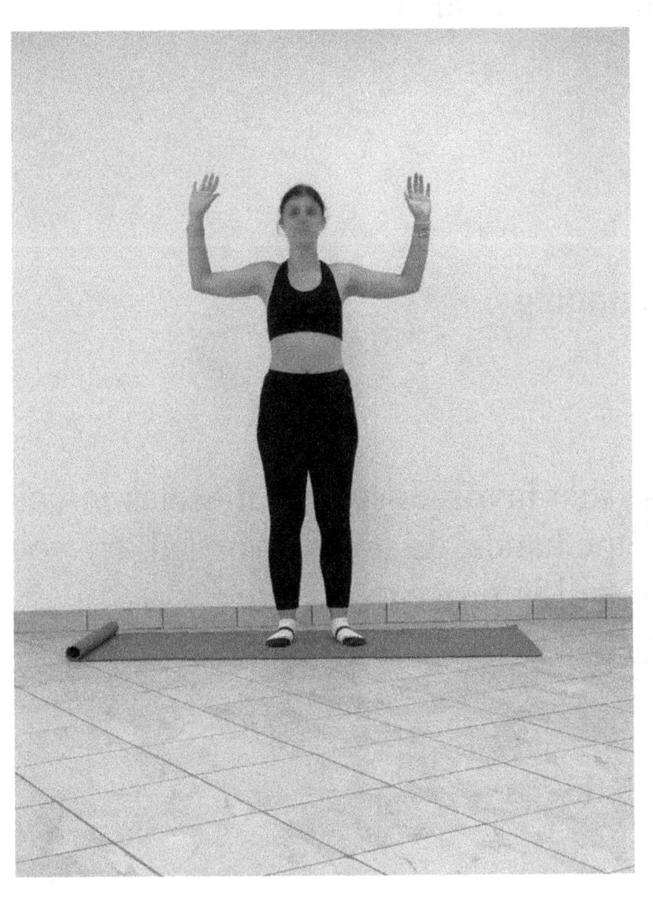

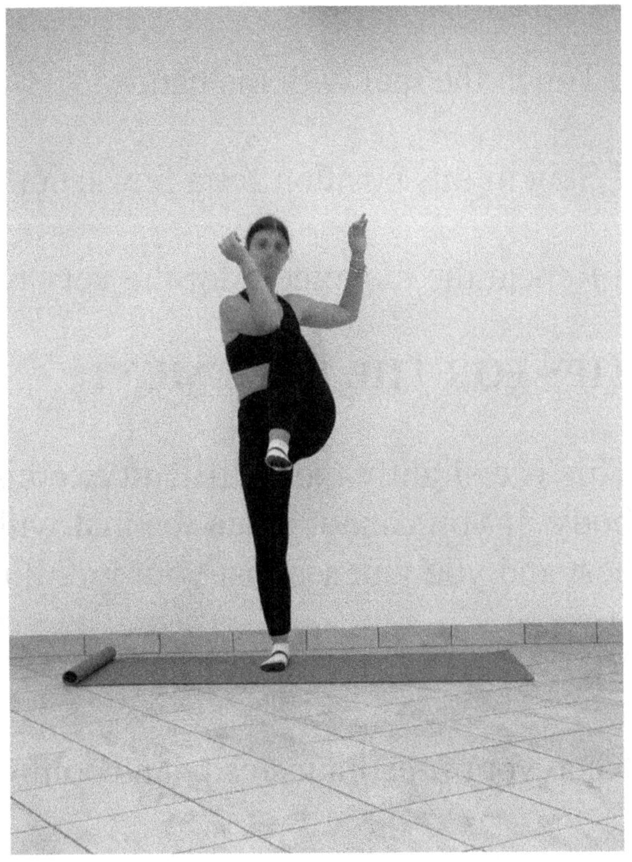

8 – BACK STRENGTHENING

BENEFITS:

- spinal muscles relaxation
- coordination improvement

HOW TO PERFORM THE EXERCISE

1 Place yourself at the center of the mat with the legs apart

2 Raise the arms by keeping them straight

3 Raise the head, looking at the ceiling

4 Spread the arms out to the side, bending down

5 Keep the legs semi-stretched and your abdominals well-contracted

6 Touch the mat with the hands

7 Stay in this position for a few seconds

8 Repeat the movement for the very beginning

TIPS FOR THE MOVEMENT

This is a slightly more difficult exercise that involves several muscles in your body. If you cannot touch the mat with the hands, do not be worried, try your best and you will see that your mobility will improve over time.

BREATHING INDICATIONS

Keep your breathing steady and controlled.

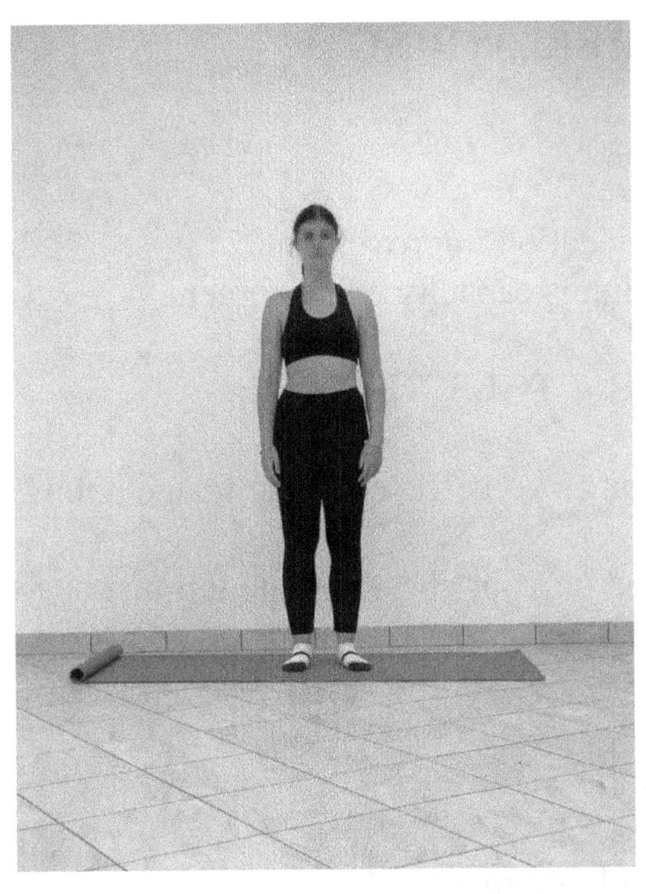

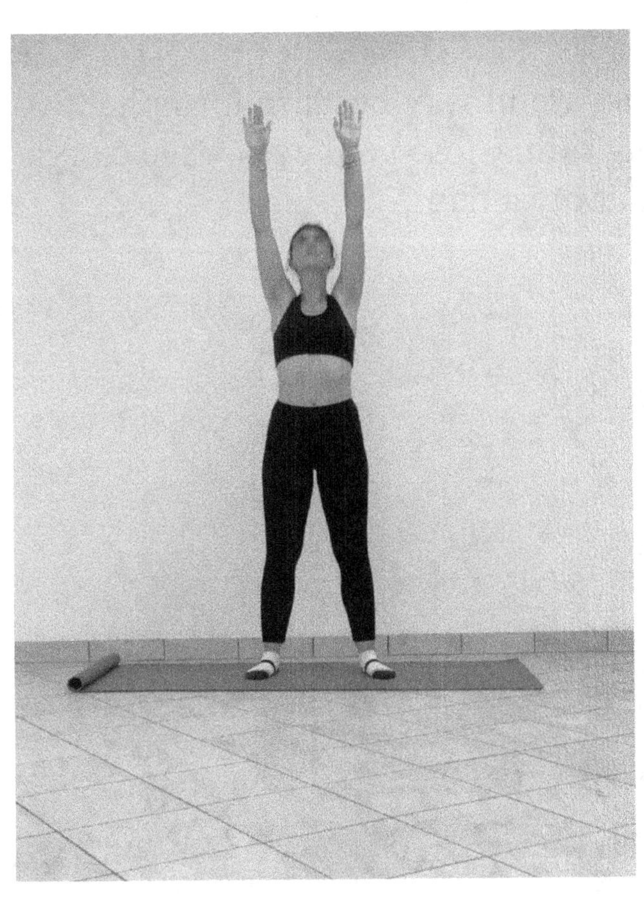

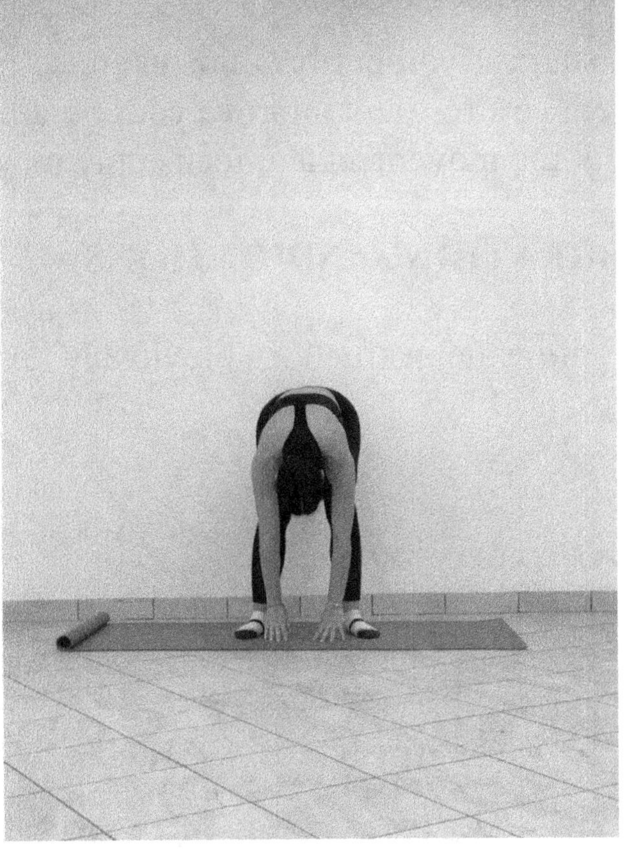

9 – SEATED DEEP BREATHING

BENEFITS:

- mind-body connection improvement
- breathing and lungs capacity enhancement

HOW TO PERFORM THE EXERCISE

1 Sit down on the mat as you can see in the image below

2 Place the right hand on your chest and the left one on your abdomen

3 Take a deep breath

4 Exhale and repeat the exercise

TIPS FOR THE MOVEMENT

I suggest you perform this exercise in a careful way because it can help you reduce stress and improve your breathing skill. Close your eyes when carrying out the movement and focus only on your breathing.

BREATHING INDICATIONS

Follow the instructions previously described.

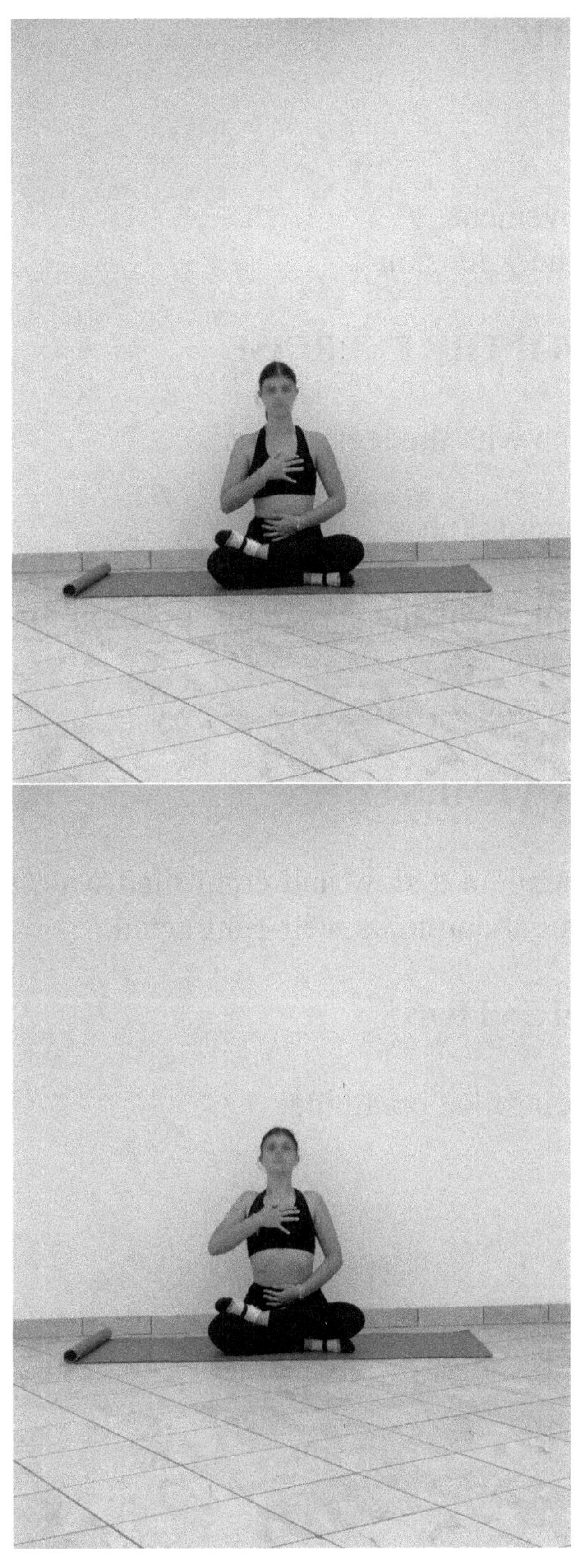

10 – NECK ROTATION

BENEFITS:

- mobility improvement
- elimination of neck tension

HOW TO PERFORM THE EXERCISE

1 Sit down on the map with the legs crossed

2 Place the hands on your knees

3 Rotate the head to the right and stay in this position for a few seconds

4 Make the same movement on the left side

TIPS FOR THE MOVEMENT

Conduct the movements in a slow and controlled way, always keeping your back straight and your abdominals well-contracted.

BREATHING INDICATIONS

Keep a steady and controlled breathing.

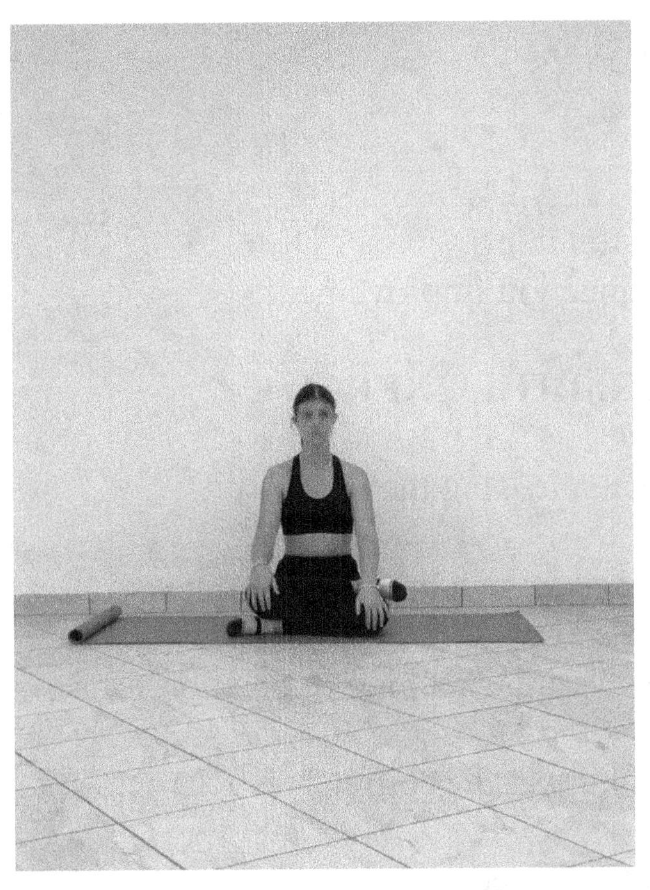

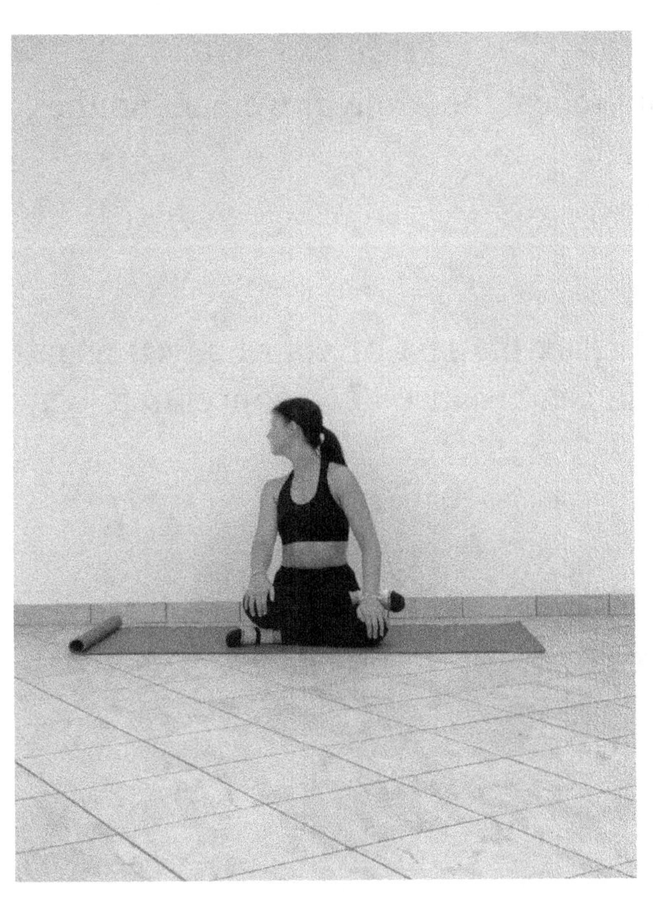

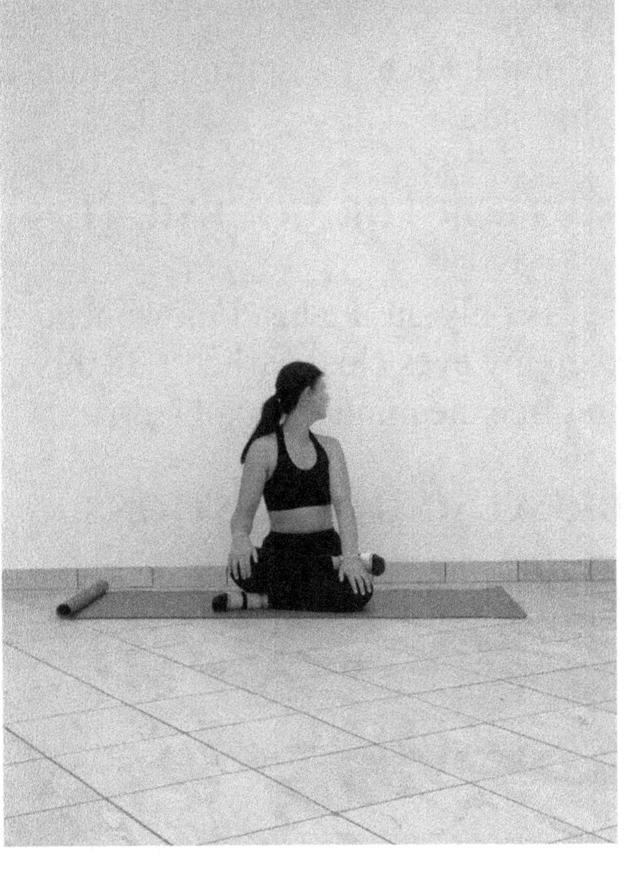

11 – NECK FLEXION

BENEFITS:

- neck muscles stretching
- mind-body connection improvement

HOW TO PERFORM THE EXERCISE

1 Sit down on the mat, crossing the legs

2 Relax the body, placing the hands on your knees

3 Bend the head downwards, keeping in position for 3 seconds

4 Raise the head, looking at the ceiling

5 Keep the position for 3 seconds

6 Come back to the starting position and repeat the same movement on the other side

TIPS FOR THE MOVEMENT

Focus only on the head movement and relax the rest of your body. I usually keep my eyes closed when I do this exercise, because I can concentrate better and free the mind from all worries.

BREATHING INDICATIONS

Keep a steady and controlled breathing.

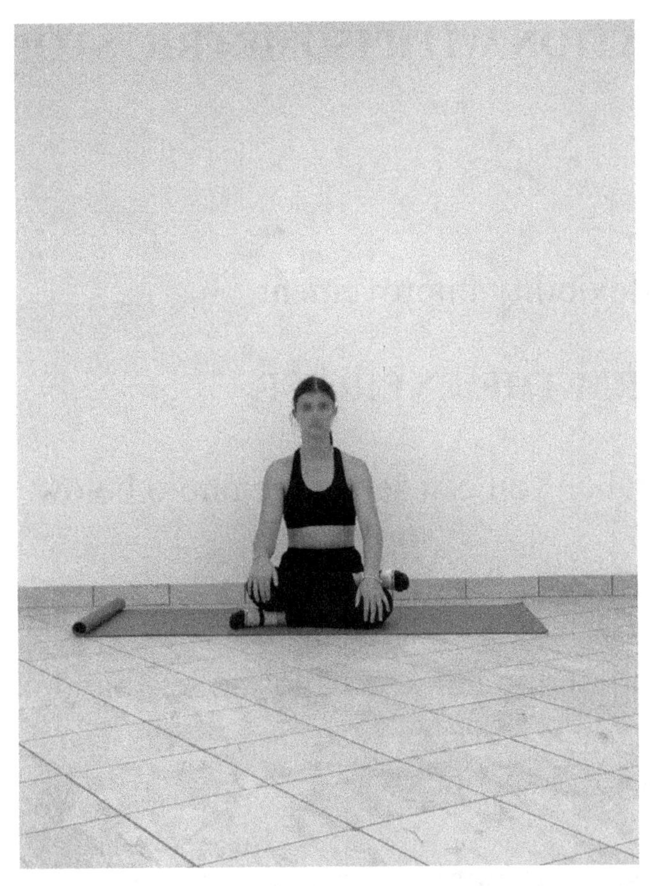

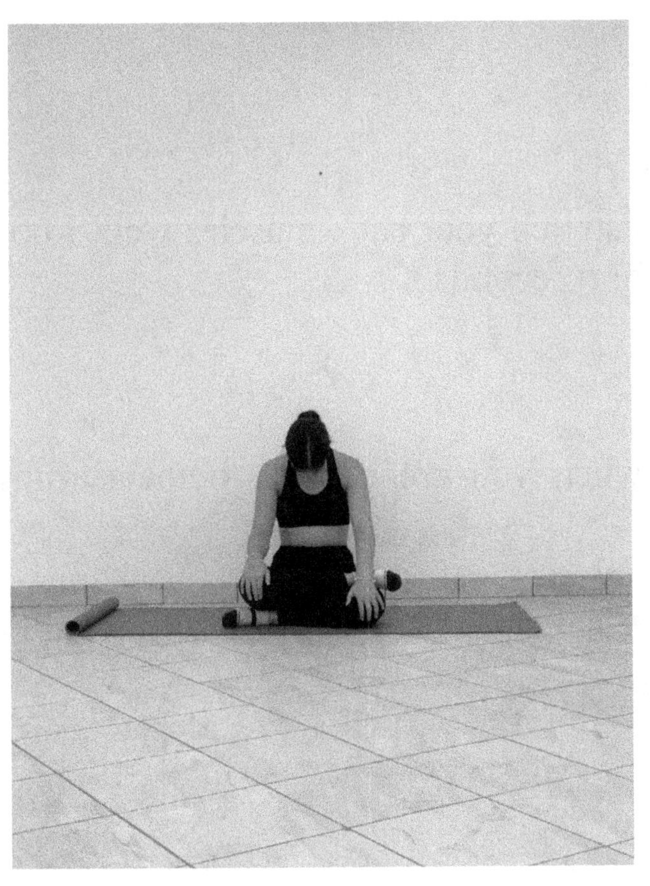

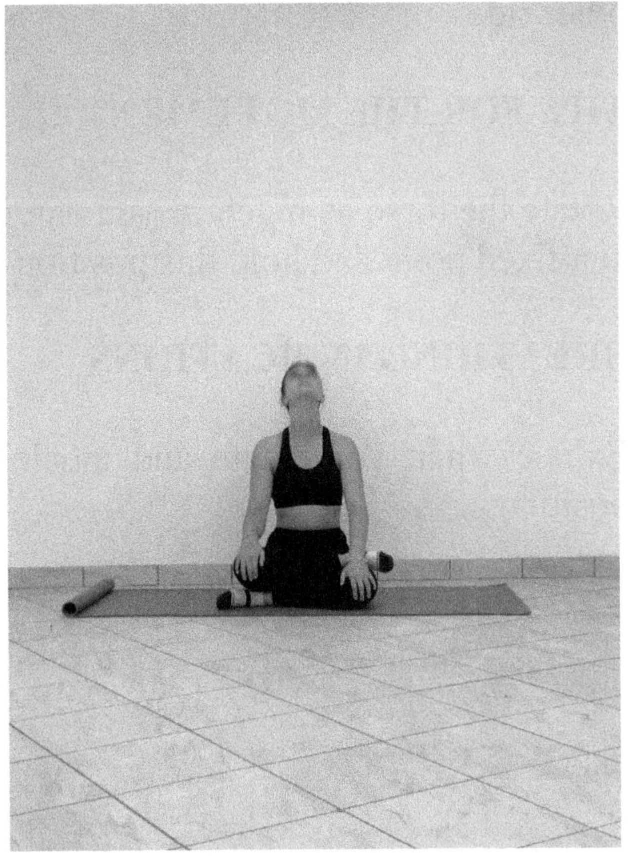

12 - TORSO ROTATION WITH ISOMETRIC STOP

BENEFITS:

- back stretching
- mobility and flexibility improvement

HOW TO PERFORM THE EXERCISE

1 Sit down on the mat as you can see in the photo below

2 Rotate your torso to the left side

3 Place the right hand on the left knee and the left hand on the floor

4 Keep this position for 5 seconds

5 Come back to the starting position, repeating the same movement on the other side

TIPS FOR THE MOVEMENT

Rotate the torso as much as you can to stretch your back muscles well. Look at a fixed point and hold this position for 5 seconds.

BREATHING INDICATIONS

Exhale when you rotate and inhale when you come back to the starting position.

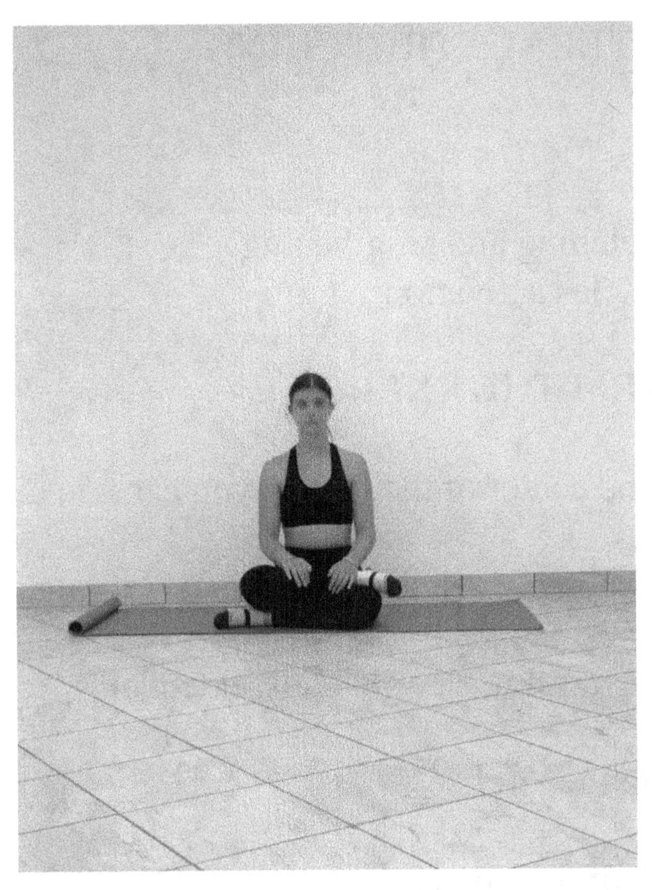
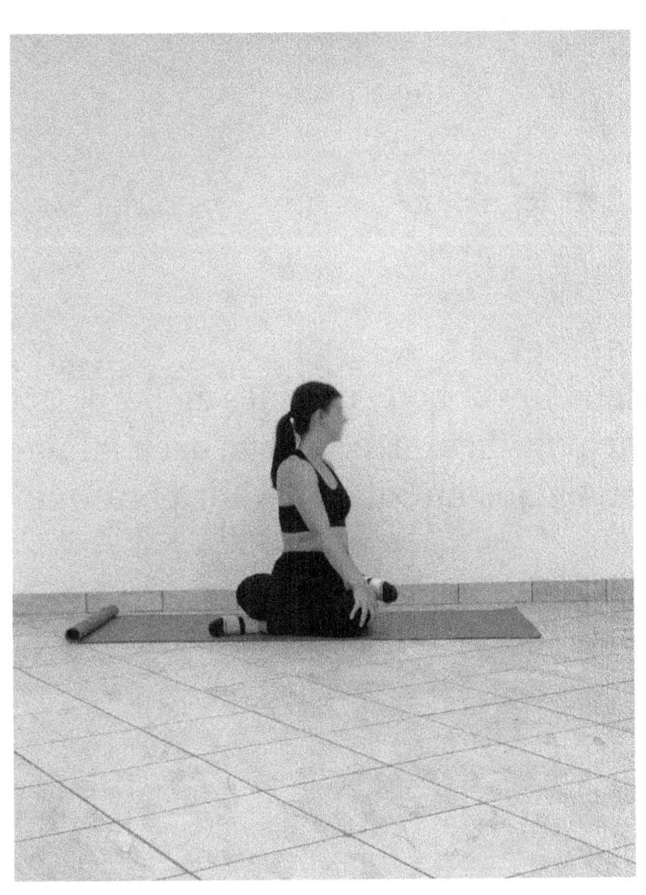
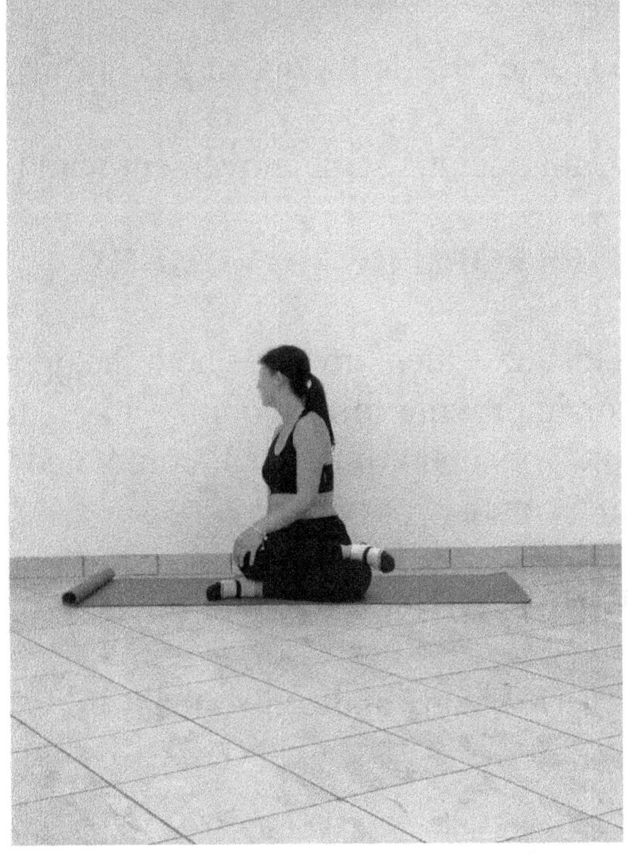

13 - LEGS UNILATERAL STRETCHING

BENEFITS:

- hamstrings stretching and lengthening
- stabilizing muscles activation

HOW TO PERFORM THE EXERCISE

1 Place yourself at the center of the mat as you can see in the image below

2 Put the hands on the mat, keeping the arms well-straight

3 Spread the right leg until it is completely extended

4 Rest the gluteus on the left heel

5 Keep the position for 5 seconds

6 Come back to the starting position

7 Conduct the same movement with the left leg

TIPS FOR THE MOVEMENT

This movement involves both the upper and lower body muscles and is perfect for improving joint mobility and lengthening them. Keep your back straight and your abdominals well-contracted to avoid losing balance while performing the exercise.

BREATHING INDICATIONS

Keep a steady and controlled way.

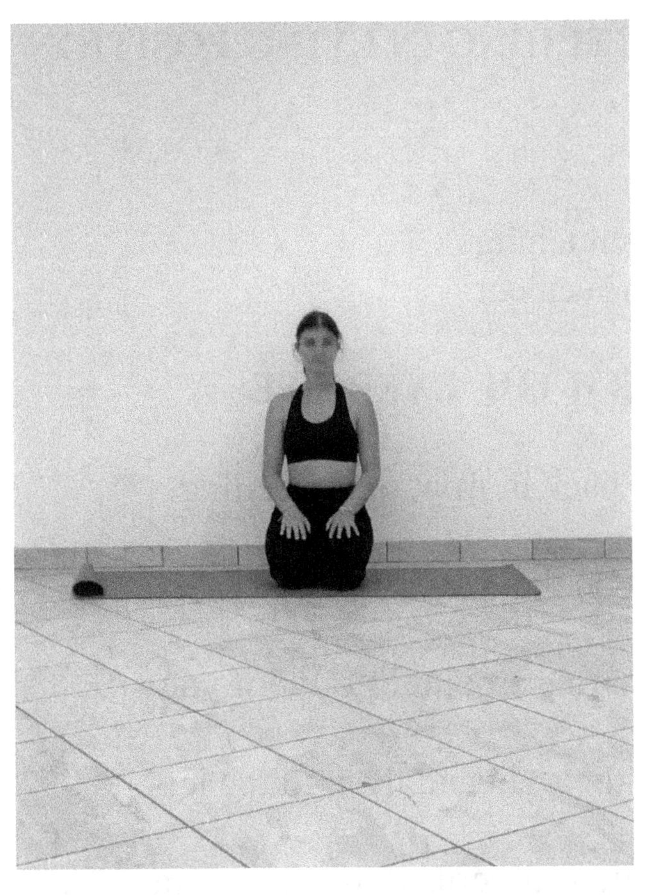

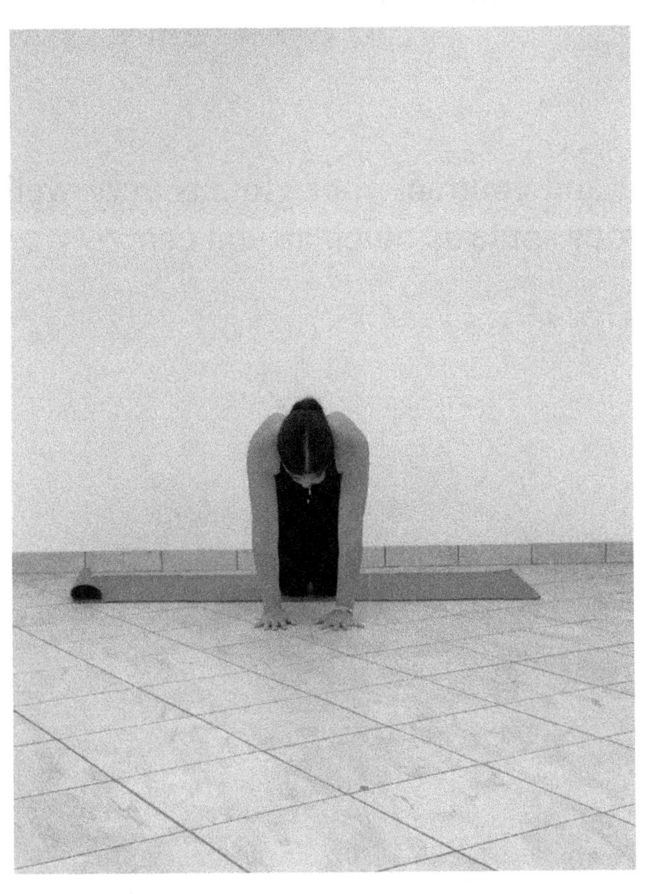

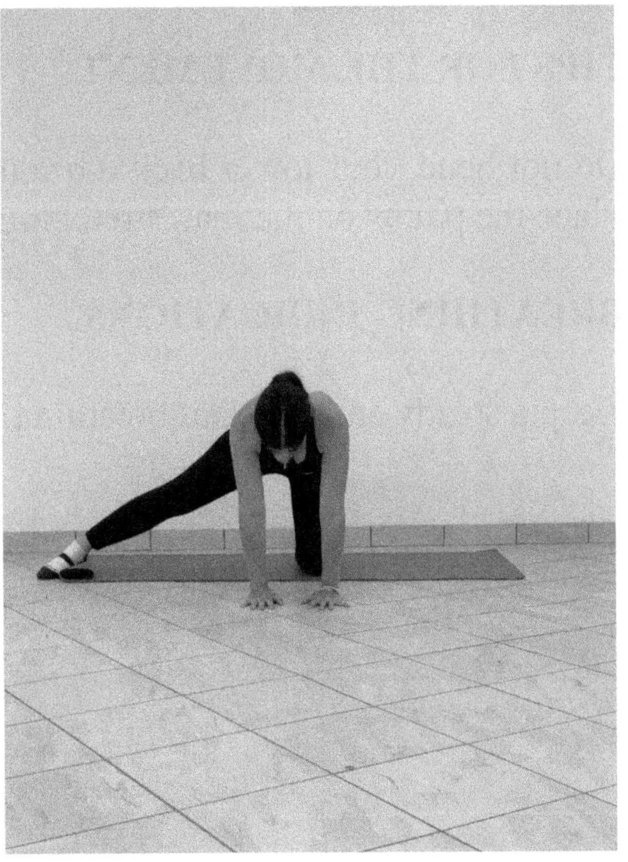

14 - STATIC STRETCHING IN LYING POSITION

BENEFITS:

- back muscles stretching
- flexibility improvement

HOW TO PERFORM THE EXERCISE

1 Lie down with the back in front of the ceiling

2 Place the forearms on the mat

3 Raise your head, staring a point in front of you

4 Rotate the head to the right and then, to the left

5 Follow the instructions described in this program

TIPS FOR THE MOVEMENT

Do not bend your lower back too much and contract your gluteus very well. Place the palms on the mat, stretching your spine as much as you can.

BREATHING INDICATIONS

Keep a steady and constant breathing.

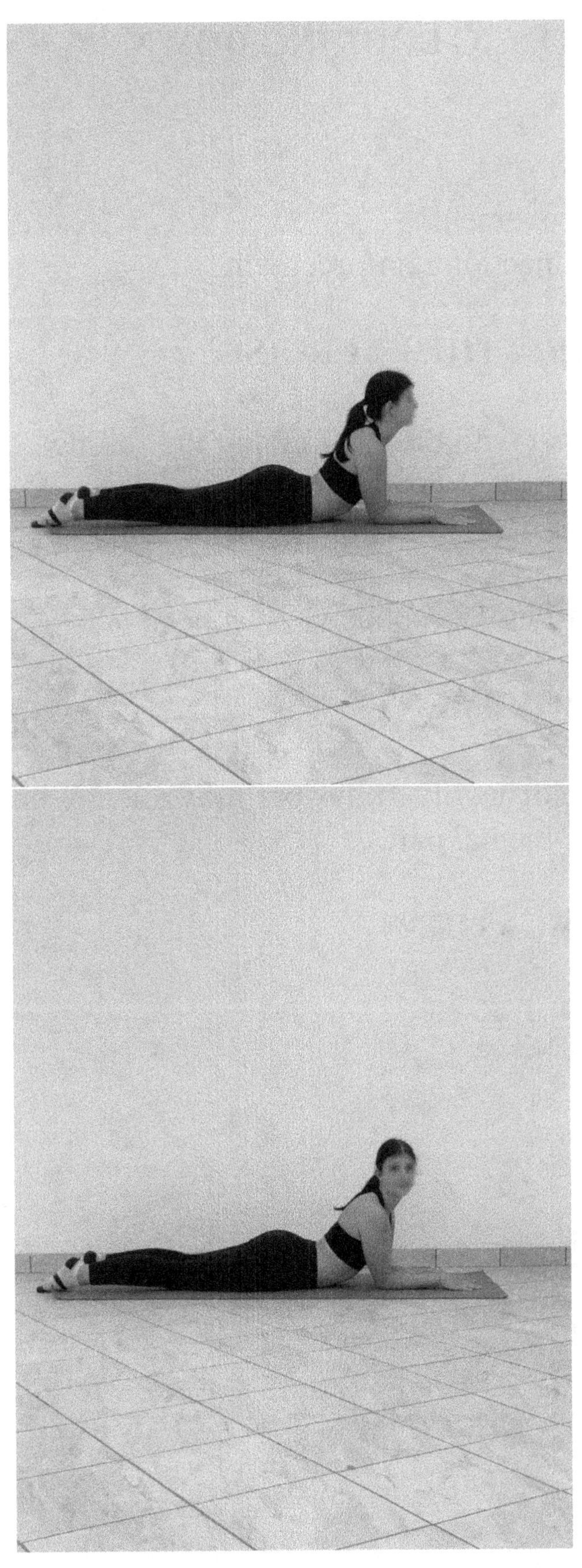

15 – DEEP BREATHING LOOKING DOWN

BENEFITS:

- breathing improvement
- mind-body connection reinforcement

HOW TO PERFORM THE EXERCISE

1 Lie down on the mat with the back facing the ceiling

2 Bend the arms, resting the forehead on your hands

3 Keep this position for 30 seconds

TIPS FOR THE MOVEMENT

This exercise does not involve physical movements, but it requires a lot of concentration on the mental part.

BREATHING INDICATIONS

Take deep breaths.

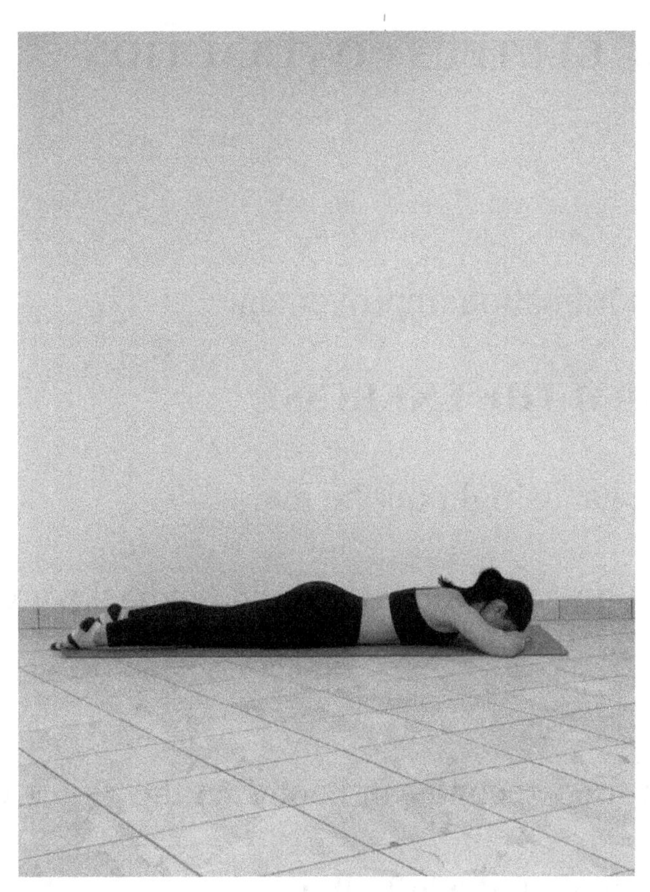

16 - UNILATERAL GLUTEUS CONTRACTION

BENEFITS:

- glutes toning
- balance and coordination improvement

HOW TO PERFORM THE EXERCISE

1 Rest you knee and hands right on the mat

2 Keep the arms straight, extending the right leg backwards

3 Raise the left arm

4 Hold this position for 3 seconds and contract the glutes very well

5 Touch the right knee with the left elbow

6 Repeat the same movement on the other side

TIPS FOR THE MOVEMENT

Keep your abdominal muscles well-contracted and your back straight during the entire exercise. Try never to lose your balance, by focusing on glutes contraction.

BREATHING INDICATIONS

Inhale when you lift your leg and exhale when you touch your elbow up to your knee.

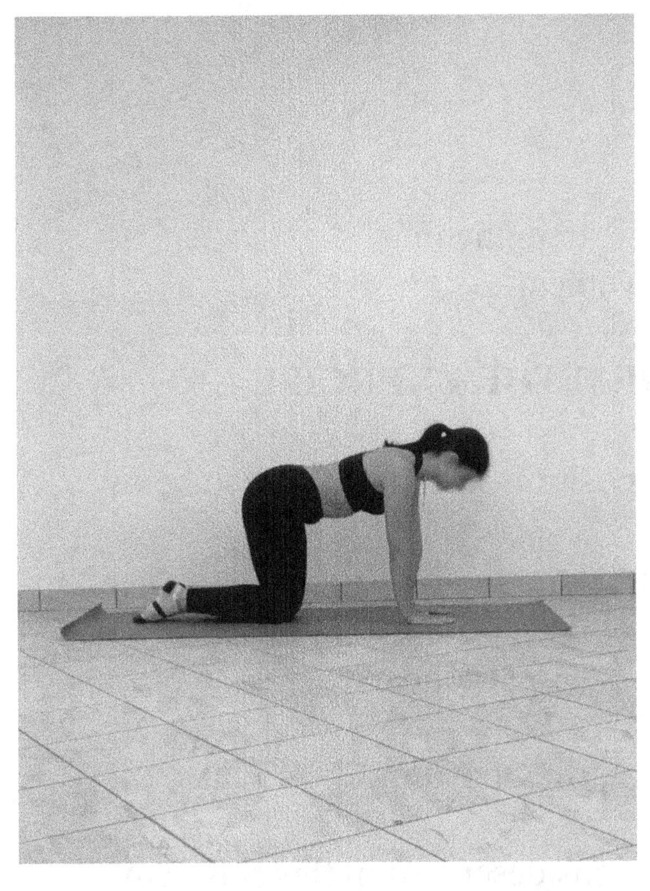

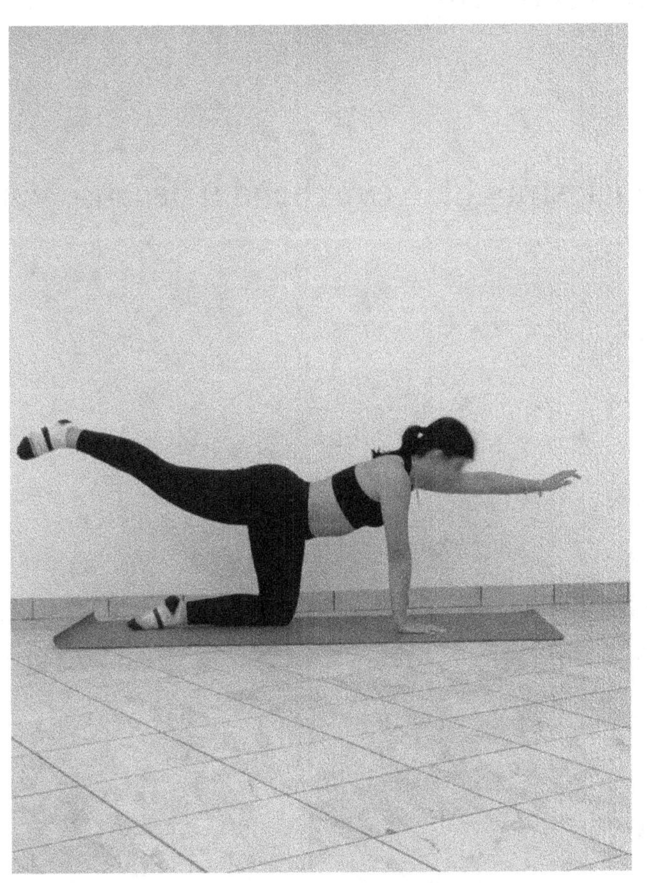

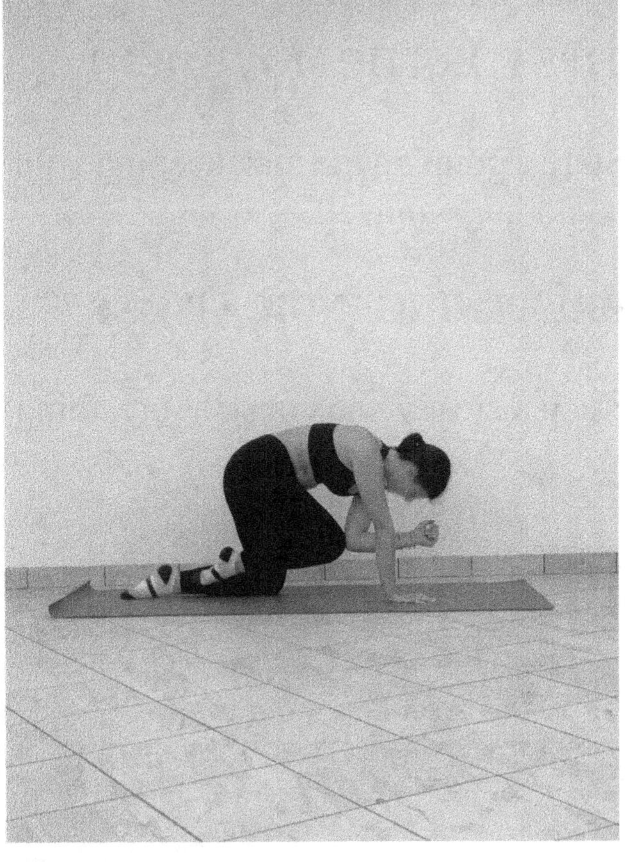

17 - PLANK

BENEFITS:

- abdominal wall strengthening
- balance improvement

HOW TO PERFORM THE EXERCISE

1 Place in the same position seen in the image below

2 Put the toes on the mat

3 Keep this position for 10 seconds

4 Come back to the starting position

5 Follow the instructions described in this program

TIPS FOR THE MOVEMENT

Stare a point on the mat, keeping your back straight. Never bend it because you could hurt yourself.

BREATHING INDICATIONS

Keep a steady and constant breathing.

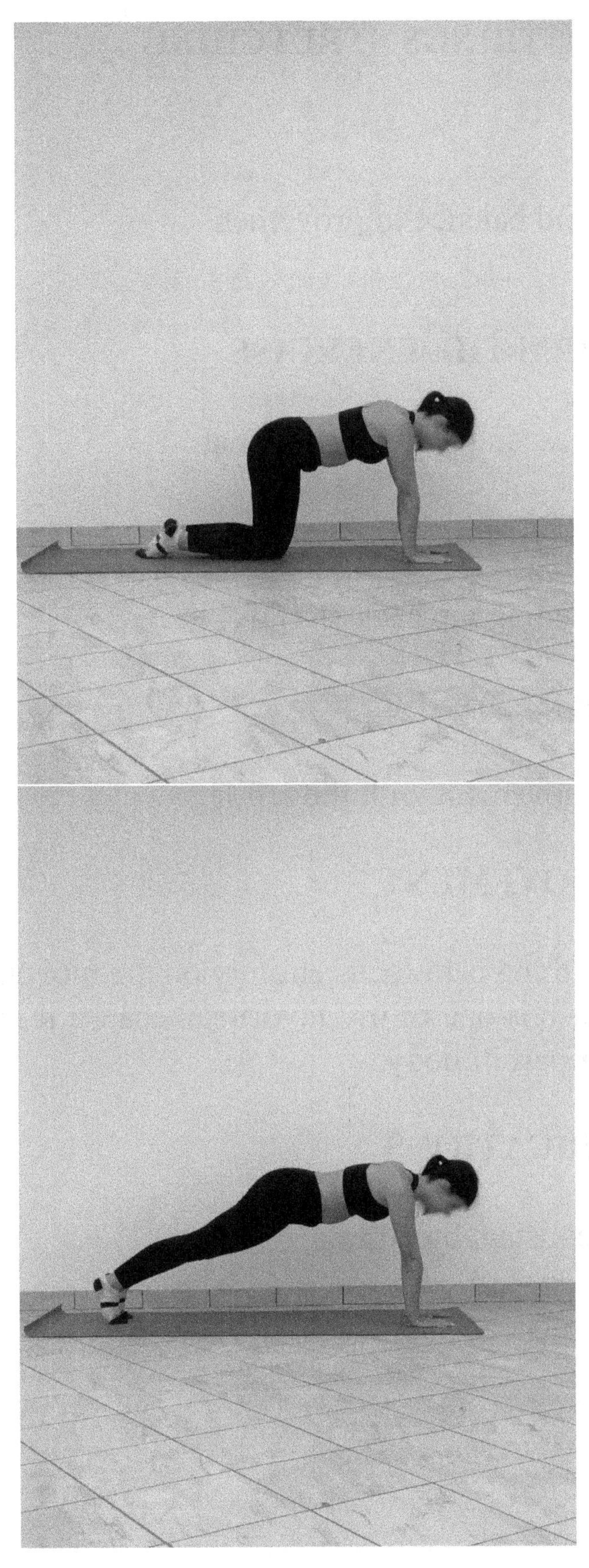

18 - STATIC HAMSTRINGS STRETCHING

BENEFITS:

- coordination and balance improvement
- glutes toning

HOW TO PERFORM THE EXERCISE

1 Place the feet, knees, and palms on the mat

2 Bring the right leg forward

3 Raise the arms, bending the back slightly

4 Keep this position for 5 seconds

5 Repeat the same movement with the left leg

TIPS FOR THE MOVEMENT

The most important thing is to focus entirely on the movement, without losing balance. This exercise is one of my favorites because it involves whether the upper and the lower part of body.

BREATHING INDICATIONS

Keep a steady and constant breathing.

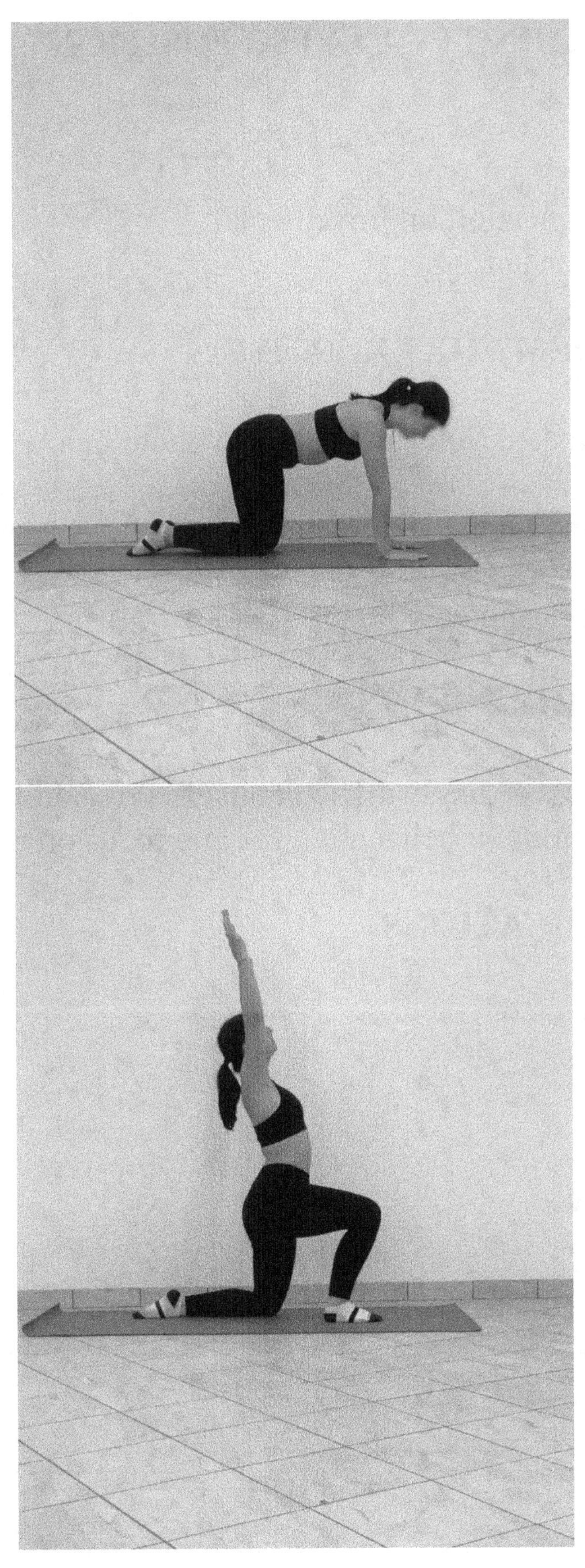

19 - DEEP BREATHING IN A LYING POSITION

BENEFITS:

- mind-body connection improvement
- lung capacity enhancement

HOW TO PERFORM THE EXERCISE

1 Lie down on the mat as you can see in the photo below

2 Place the right hand on the abdomen and the left hand on your chest

3 Close the eyes, focusing on yourself

TIPS FOR THE MOVEMENT

This exercise is not exceedingly difficult but effective. Indeed, I always include it in my workout routine. It helps me relax and focus on my goals.

BREATHING INDICATIONS

Take deep breaths.

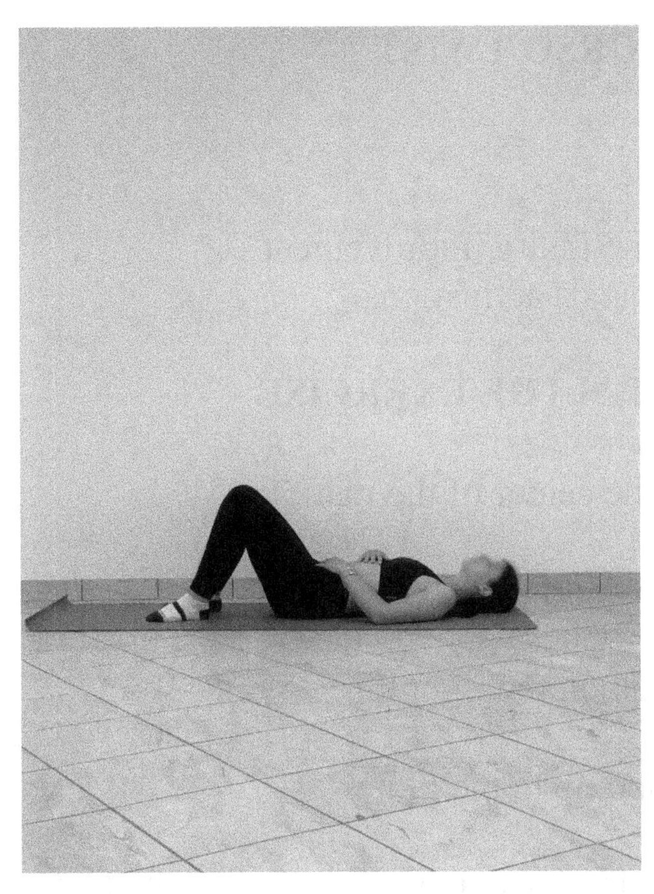

20 - STANDING TORSO TWIST

BENEFITS:

- mobility and flexibility improvement
- oblique abdominals activation

HOW TO PERFORM THE EXERCISE

1 Place yourself at the center of the mat

2 Rotate the torso to the right

3 Place your left hand on the right hip

4 Move the right hand up to the glutes

5 Keep this position for 3 seconds

6 Repeat the same movement on the other side

TIPS FOR THE MOVEMENT

Do not rotate your torso quickly, conduct the movement in a slow and controlled way, trying not to strain your lower back too much to avoid injuries and pain.

BREATHING INDICATIONS

Exhale when you rotate the torso and inhale when you come back to the starting position.

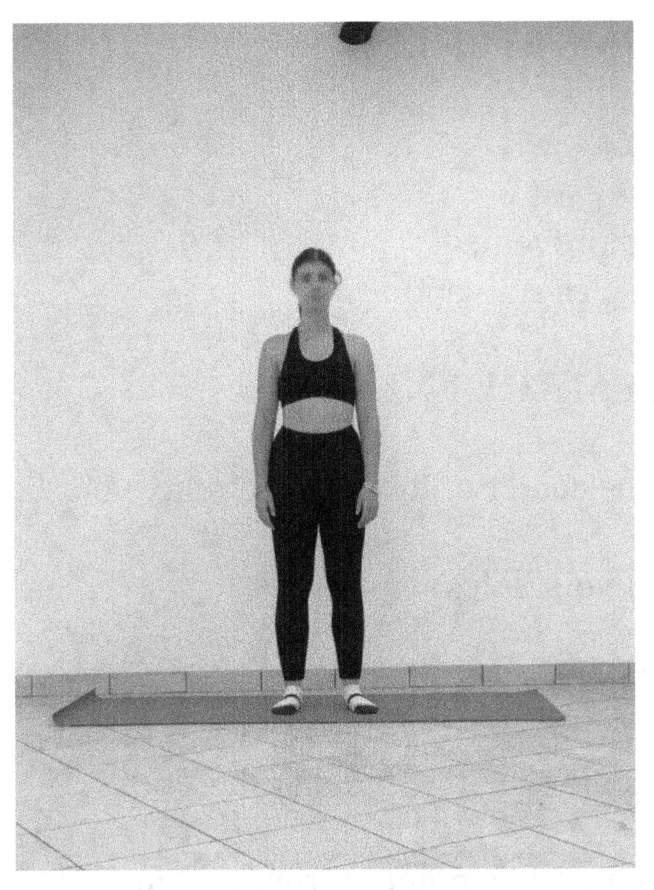

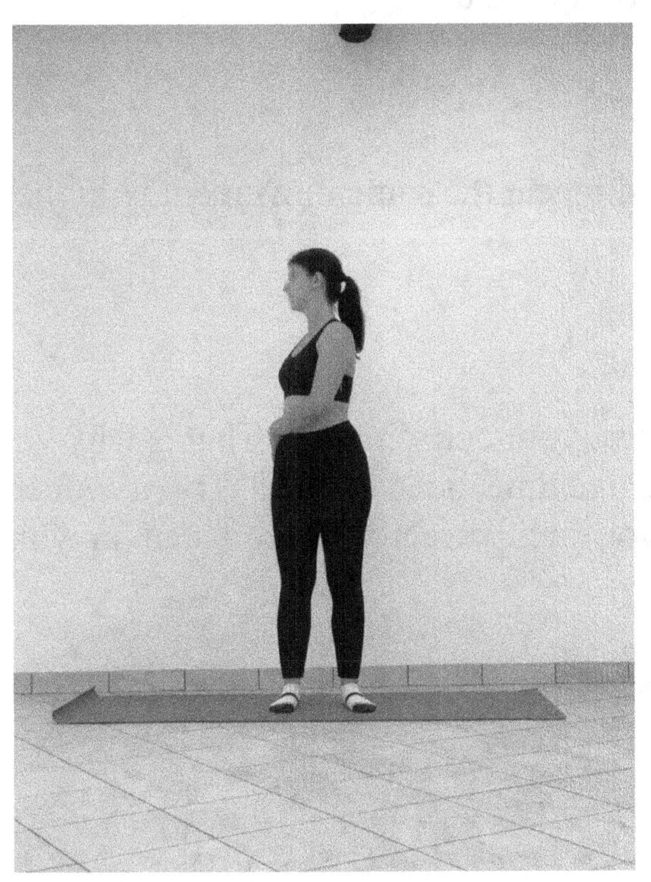

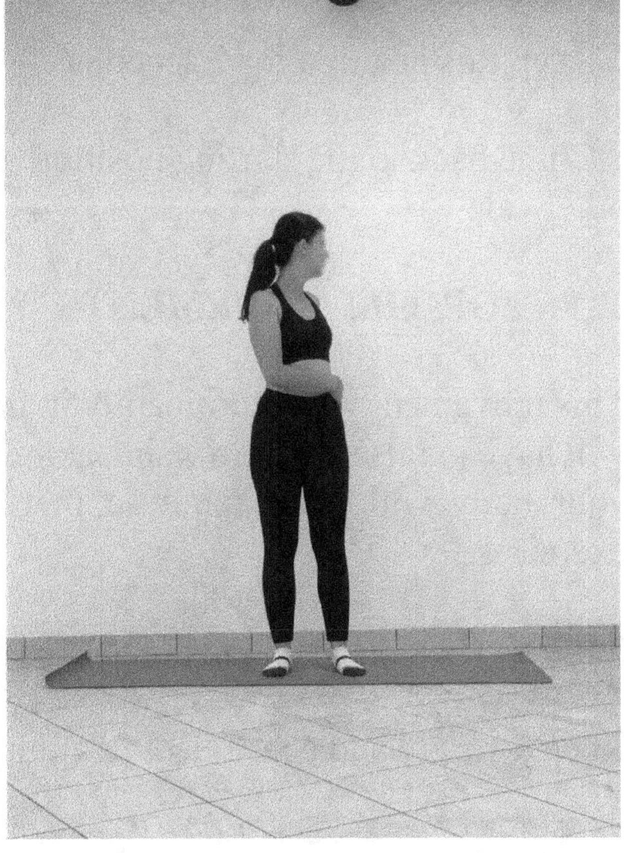

21 - LATERAL ARMS STRETCHING

BENEFITS:

- coordination improvement
- stabilizing muscles activation

HOW TO PERFORM THE EXERCISE

1 Place yourself at the center of the mat and relax your body

2 Extend the arms at your sides

3 Keep the legs and the back well-straight

4 Raise the arms, keeping them parallel to the floor

5 Bend the knees, staring at a point in front of you

6 Keep this position for 5 seconds

7 Come back to the starting position and repeat the same movement with the other side

TIPS FOR THE MOVEMENT

This movement will significantly improve your coordination. That is why you will have to raise your arms and, at the same time, bend the legs. Try to connect your body with your mind so that you are perfectly coordinated in your exercises.

BREATHING INDICATIONS

Keep a steady and controlled breathing.

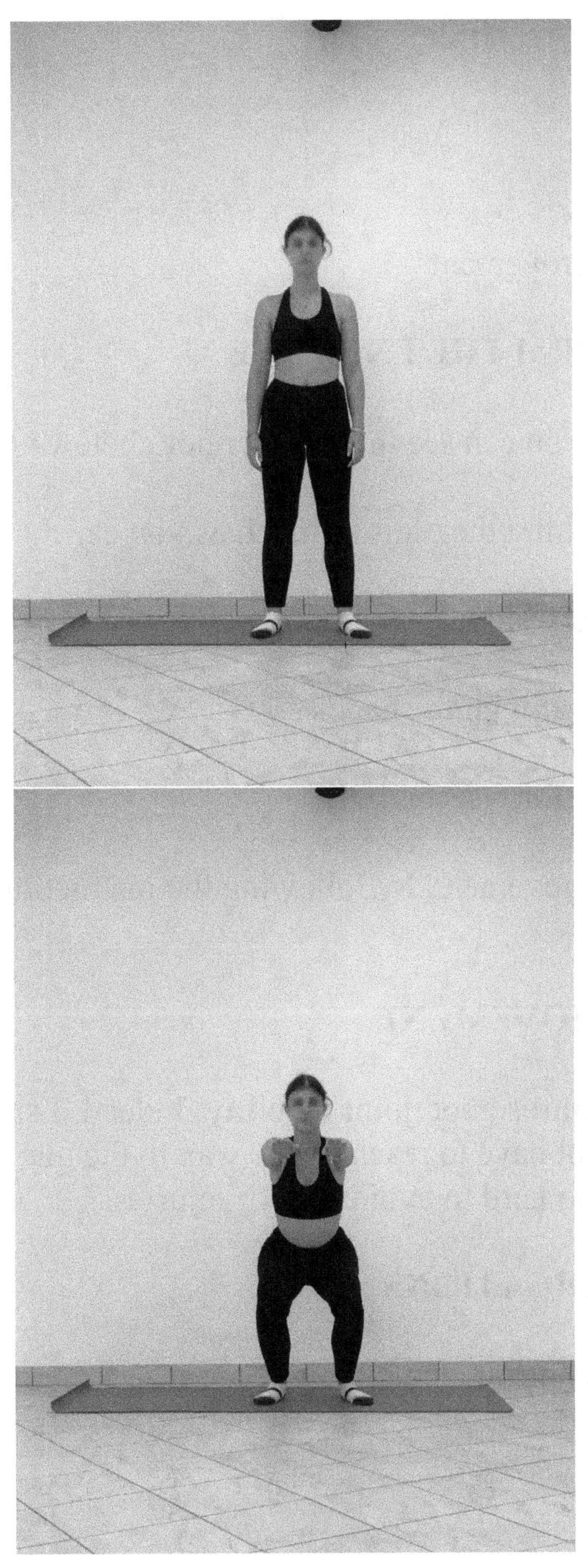

22 - TORSO STRETCHING

BENEFITS:

- back stretching
- flexibility improvement

HOW TO PERFORM THE EXERCISE

1 Place yourself as you can see in the first photo below

2 Bend down, stretching the arms as much as you can

3 Bend the knees very slightly

4 Try to touch the mat with the hands

5 Keep this position for 5 seconds

6 Repeat the same movement, by following the instructions described in this program

TIPS FOR THE MOVEMENT

This movement requires good joint mobility. Indeed, I suggest you do it very carefully. You do not have to reach all the way to the mat with your hands. Do not push yourself too hard to avoid pain or injuries.

BREATHING INDICATIONS

Keep a steady and controlled breathing.

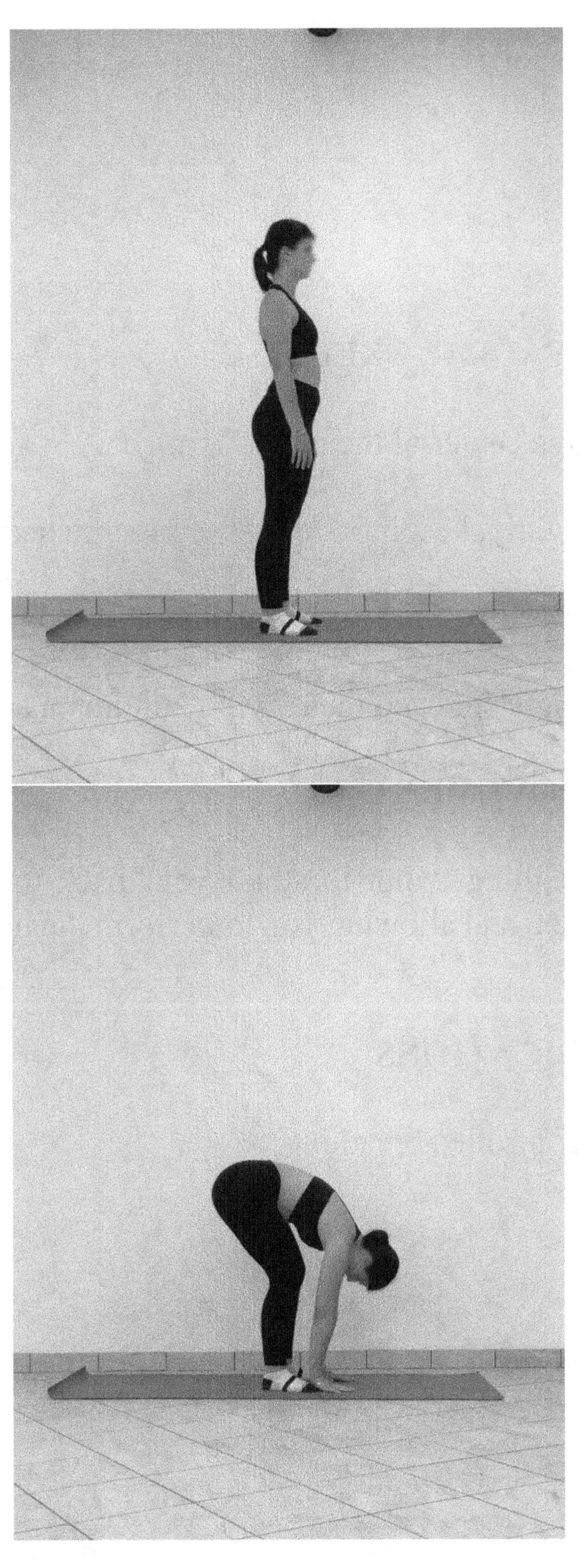

23 - DYNAMIC ROCKING

BENEFITS:

- spine stretching
- hamstrings activation

HOW TO PERFORM THE EXERCISE

1 Place yourself at the center of the mat

2 Stretch the feet slightly, keeping the legs semi-stretched

3 Bend down, by extending the arms as much as you can

4 Move first to the right side and then, to the left one in a slow way

TIPS FOR THE MOVEMENT

The most important thing is not to strain your back too much, finding the perfect rhythm for you and allowing you to perform the movement slowly and fluidly.

BREATHING INDICATIONS

Keep a steady and controlled breathing.

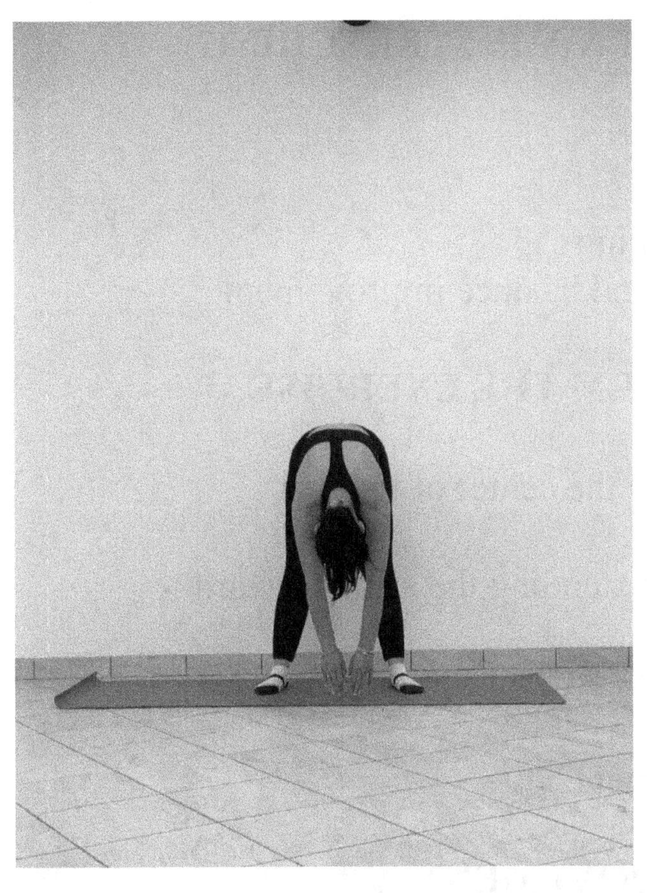

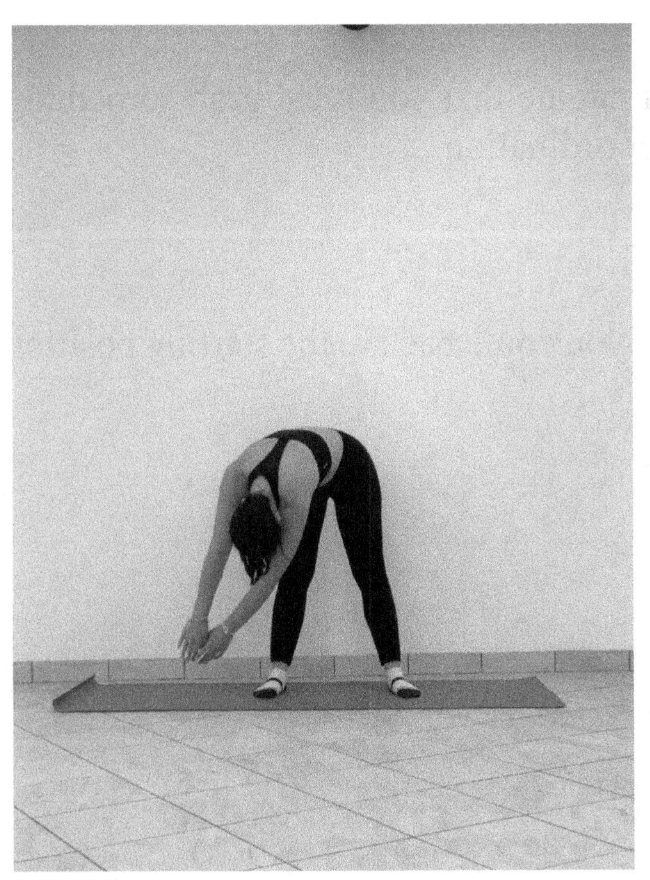

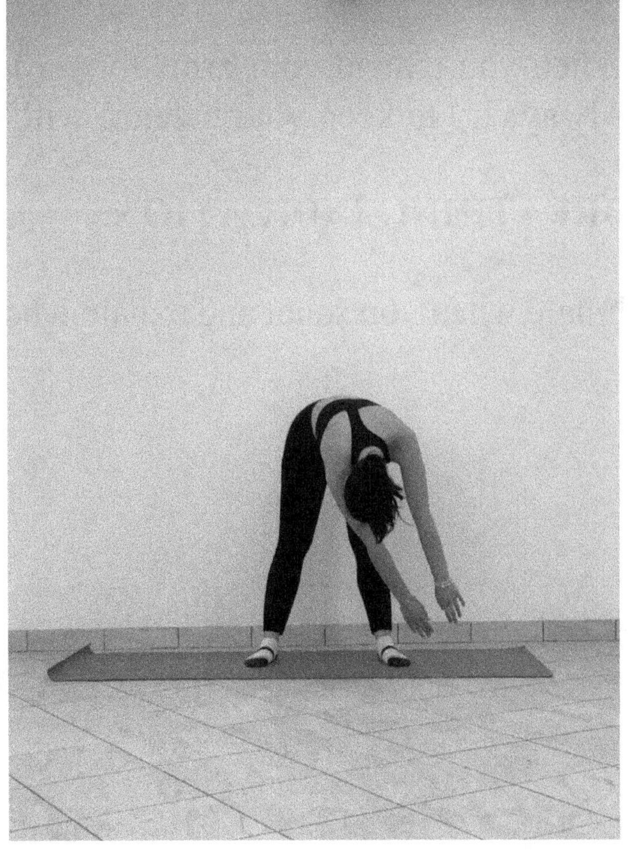

24 - SQUAT WITH ARMS STRETCHING

BENEFITS:

- quadriceps toning
- coordination and balance improvement

HOW TO PERFORM THE EXERCISE

1 Place yourself and the center of the mat

2 Perform a squat, extending the arms forward

3 Come back to the starting position

4 Repeat the movement

TIPS FOR THE MOVEMENT

When you extend your arms forward imagine that you must grab something. Always try to keep your balance with coordination.

BREATHING INDICATIONS

Inhale when you squat and exhale when you come back to the starting position.

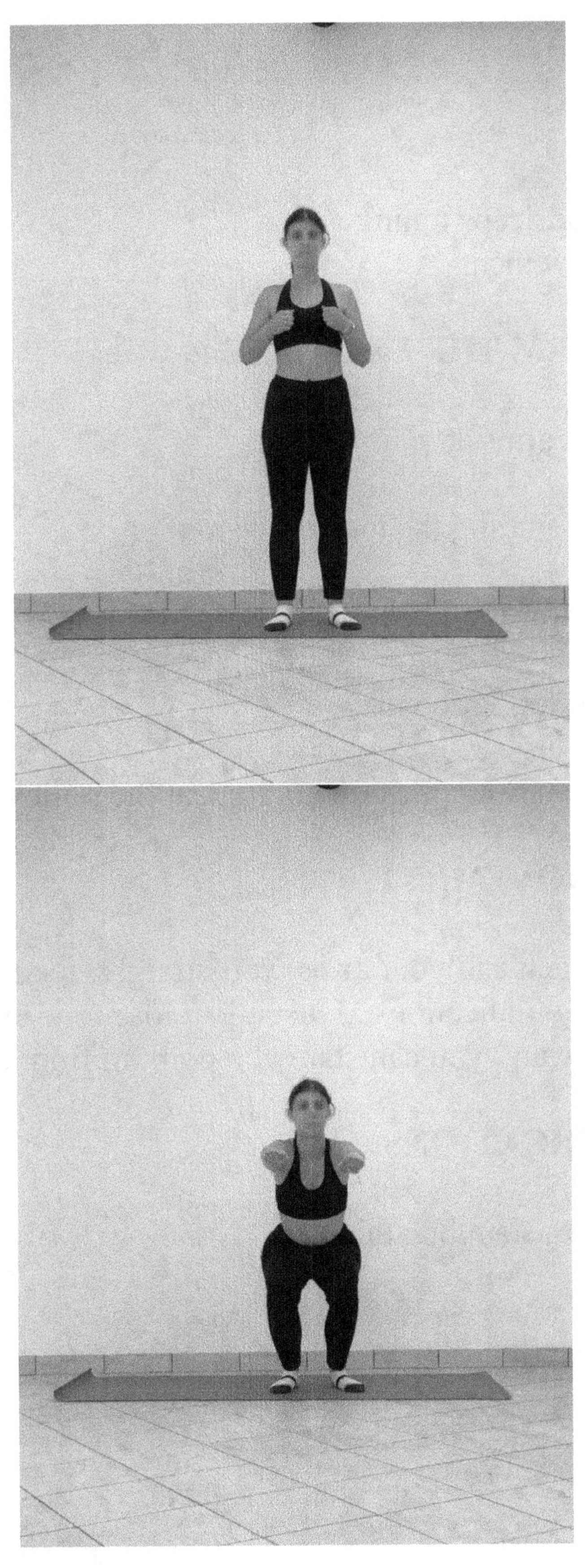

25 - STATIC SQUAT

BENEFITS:

- glutes and quadriceps toning
- balance improvement

HOW TO PERFORM THE EXERCISE

1 Place yourself and arms at your sides

2 Spread the legs by putting the toes outwards

3 Raise the arms upwards and conduct a squat

4 Keep this position for 5 seconds

5 Come back to the starting position and repeat the same movement

TIPS FOR THE MOVEMENT

Always keep your back and your arms well-straight, focusing on yourself and on correct breathing indications. I usually close my eyes when I do this exercise but, if you want, you can stare at a point in front of you.

BREATHING INDICATIONS

Keep a steady and constant breathing.

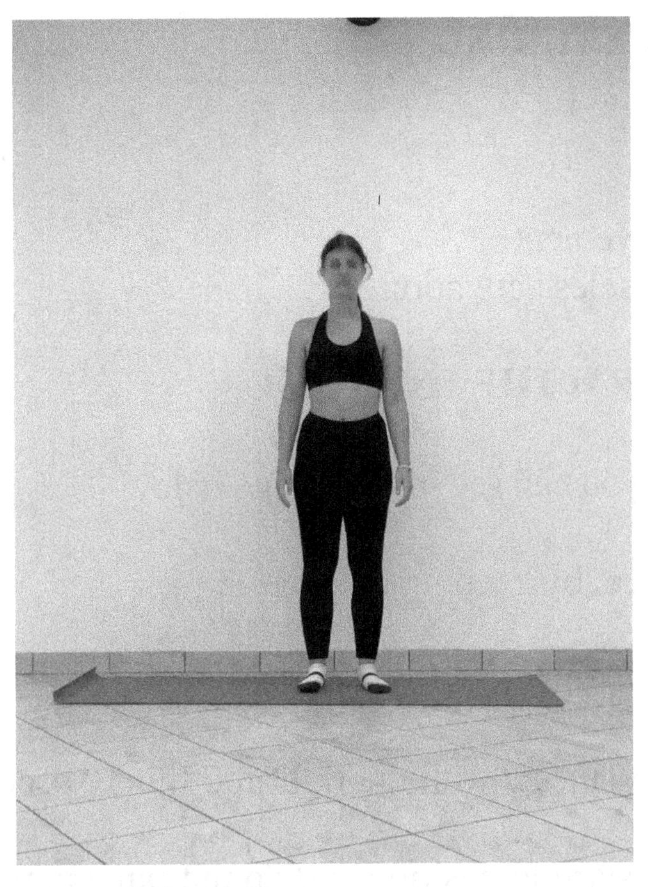

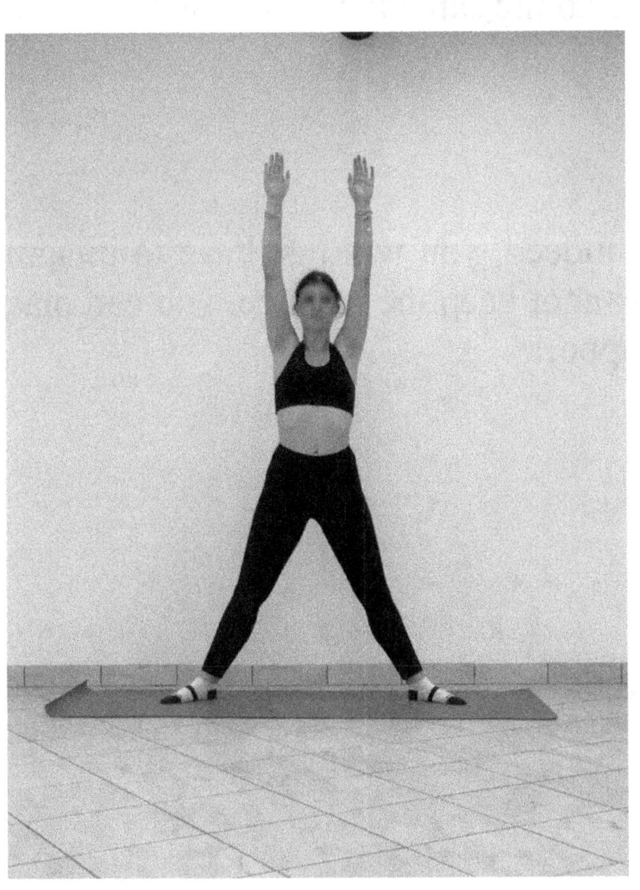

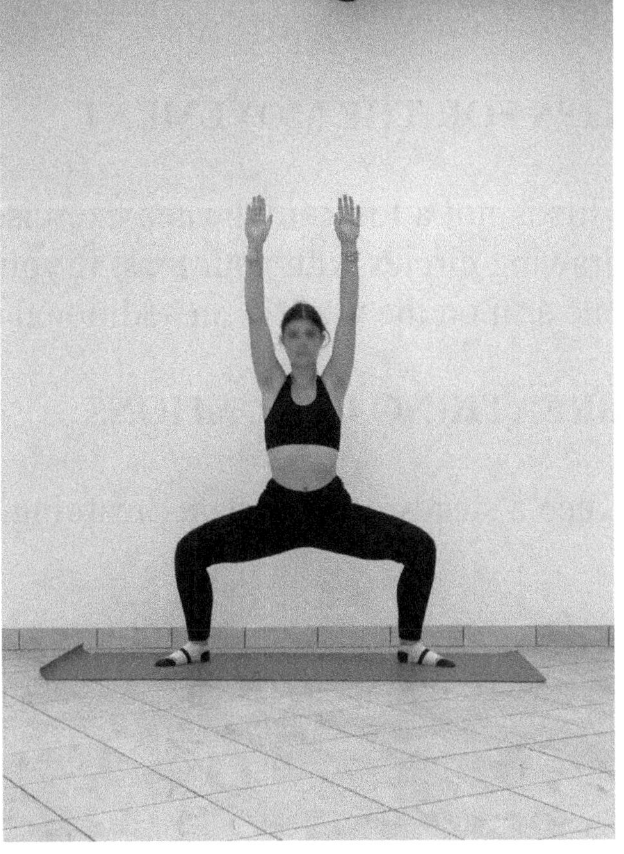

26 - CALVES STRETCHING

BENEFITS:

- balance improvement
- stabilizing muscles activation

HOW TO PERFORM THE EXERCISE

1 Place yourself as you can see in the image below

2 Raise the right knee, by keeping balance

3 Extend the arms at your sides, by maintaining the back well-straight

4 Make circular movements with the right foot for 10 seconds

5 Come back to the starting position and do the same movement with the left foot

TIPS FOR THE MOVEMENT

This is not a too complicated exercise. Indeed, you will just have to imagine drawing circles with your toes. If you cannot keep the balance, you can place one arm on the wall for an additional support.

BREATHING INDICATIONS

Keep a steady and constant breathing.

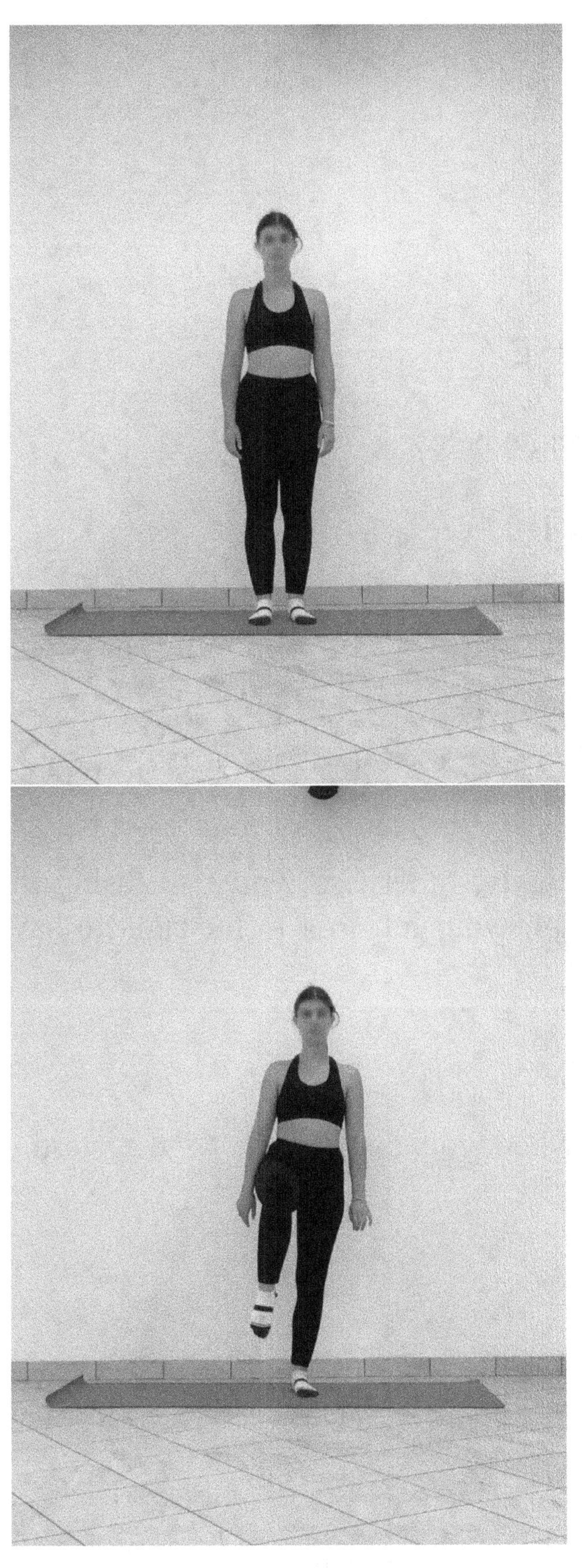

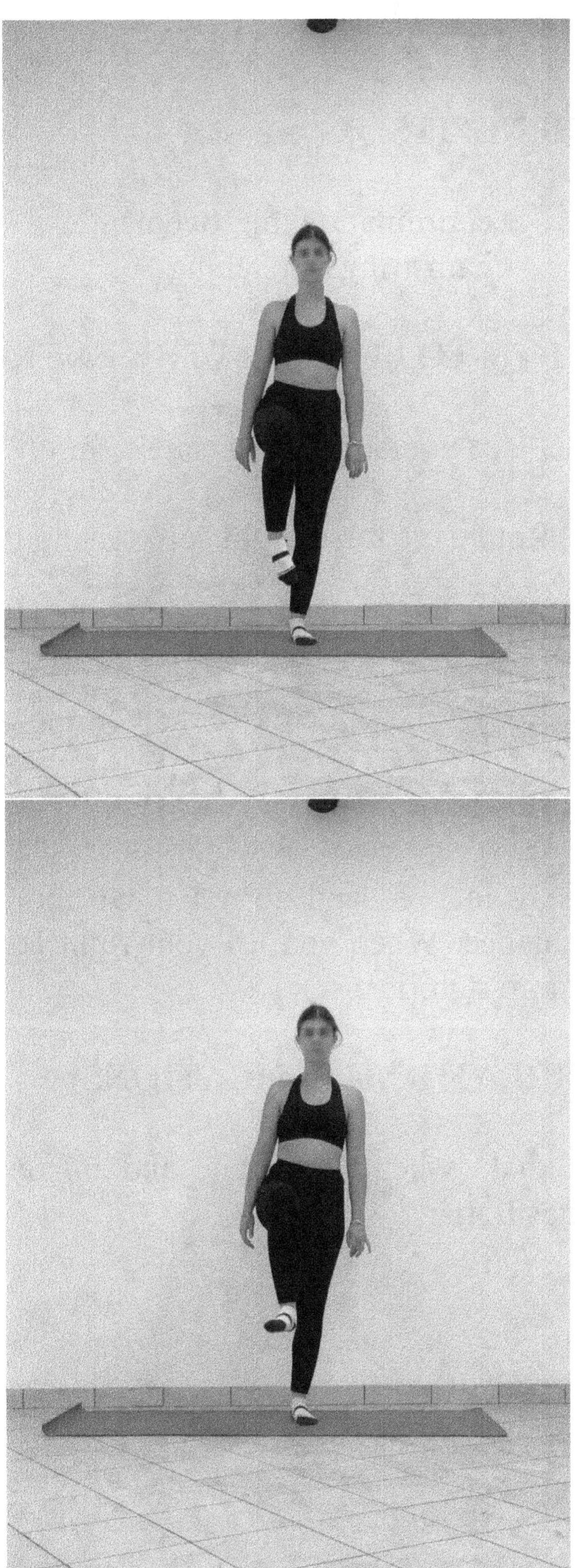

27 - DYNAMIC WALKING

BENEFITS:

- coordination improvement
- hamstrings stretching

HOW TO PERFORM THE EXERCISE

1 Place yourself as you can see in the photo below

2 Rotate the torso to the left, raising the left knee

3 Come back to the starting position

4 Repeat the same movement on the other side

TIPS FOR THE MOVEMENT

Stay focused and do not move too quickly; otherwise, you risk losing the balance. When you lift your right leg, put your left foot to the right to have more stability.

BREATHING INDICATIONS

Exhale when you rotate and inhale when you come back to the starting position.

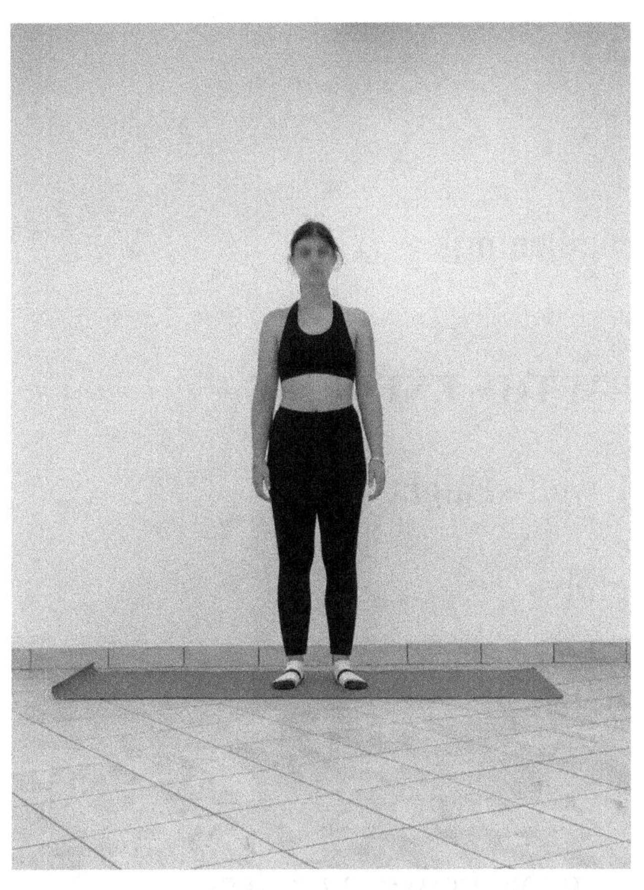

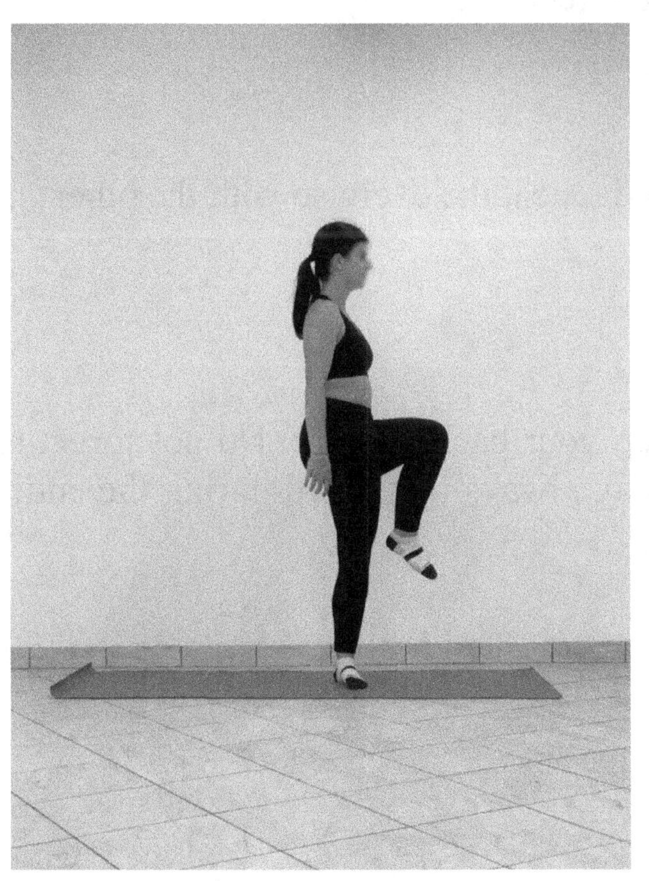

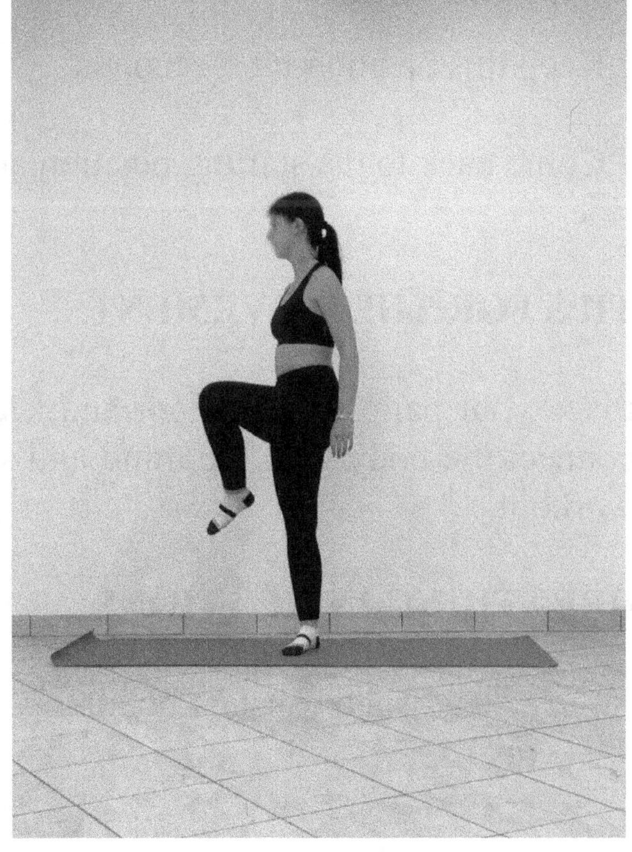

28 – STATIC SQUAT

BENEFITS:

- quadriceps strengthening
- glutes toning

HOW TO PERFORM THE EXERCISE

1 Place with the back well-straight

2 Spread the legs slightly

3 Point the toes outwards

4 Do a squat

5 Place the hands on the mat between the feet

6 Keep this position for 5 seconds

7 Come back to the starting position and repeat the exercise with the other side

TIPS FOR THE MOVEMENT

Place your palms on the floor and keep your back straight. Do not forget to connect the body with the mind and stay always motivated during the entire workout.

BREATHING INDICATIONS

Keep a steady and constant breathing.

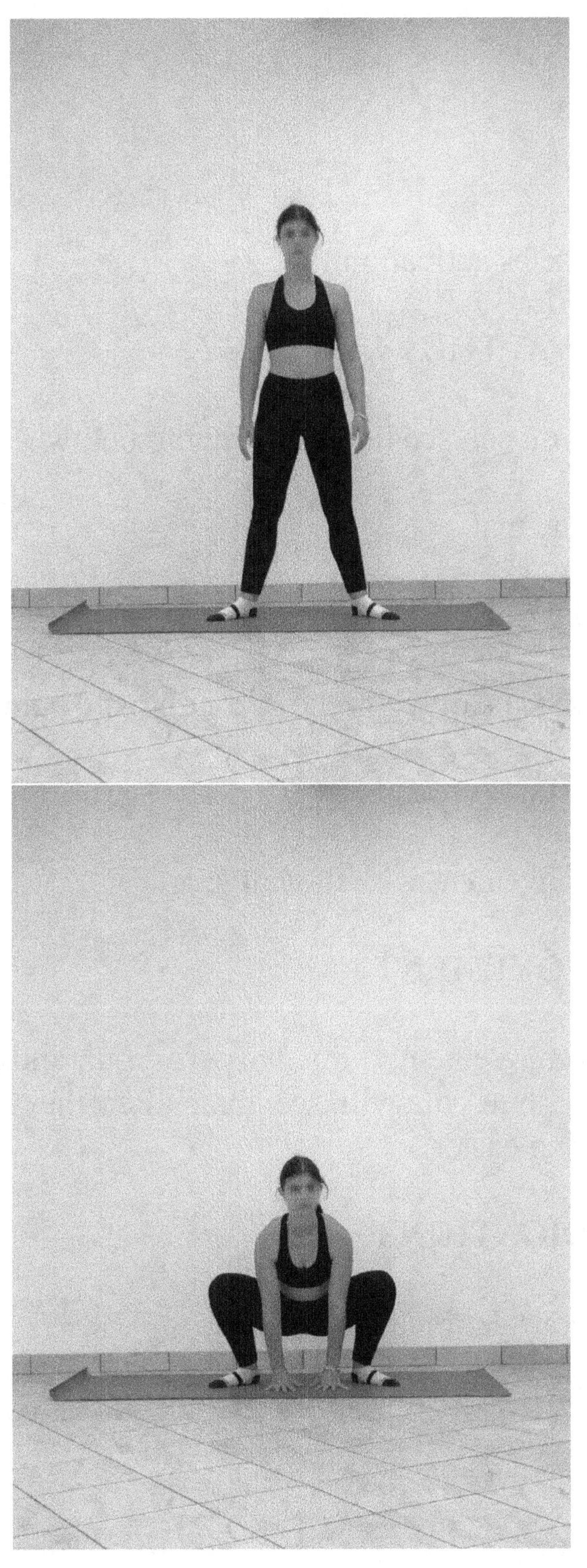

29 - ROCKING

BENEFITS:

- balance improvement
- stabilizing muscles activation

HOW TO PERFORM THE EXERCISE

1 Place yourself as you can see in the first photo below

2 Put the palms on the mat

3 Bend slightly to the right side

4 Place the hands as you can see in the second image below

5 Keep this position for 3 seconds

6 Repeat the same movement with the left side

TIPS FOR THE MOVEMENT

I recently added this movement to my daily workout, and I love it! It is a little complicated at first, but you will see that, after the first few repetitions, everything will getting easier.

BREATHING INDICATIONS

Keep a steady and constant breathing.

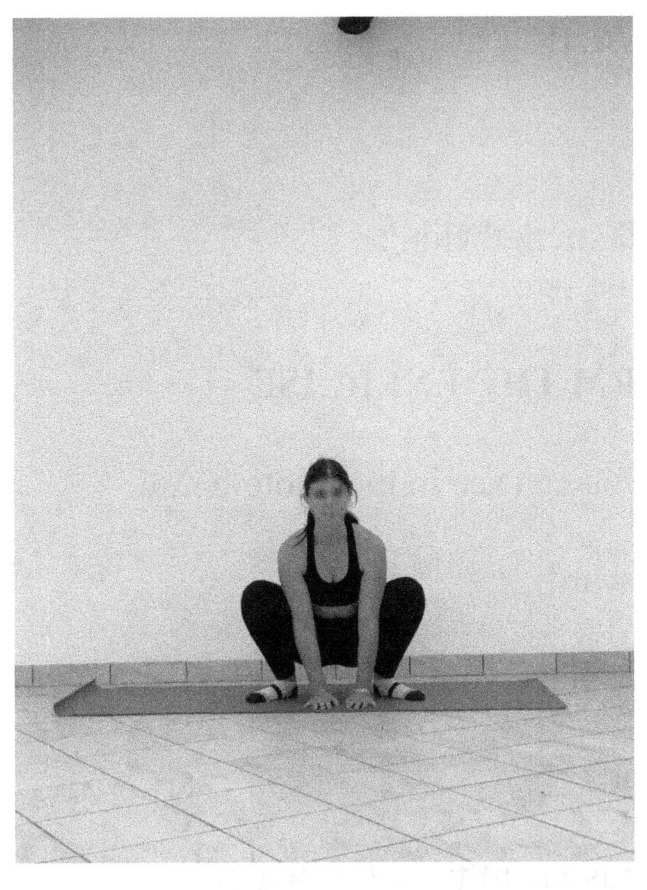

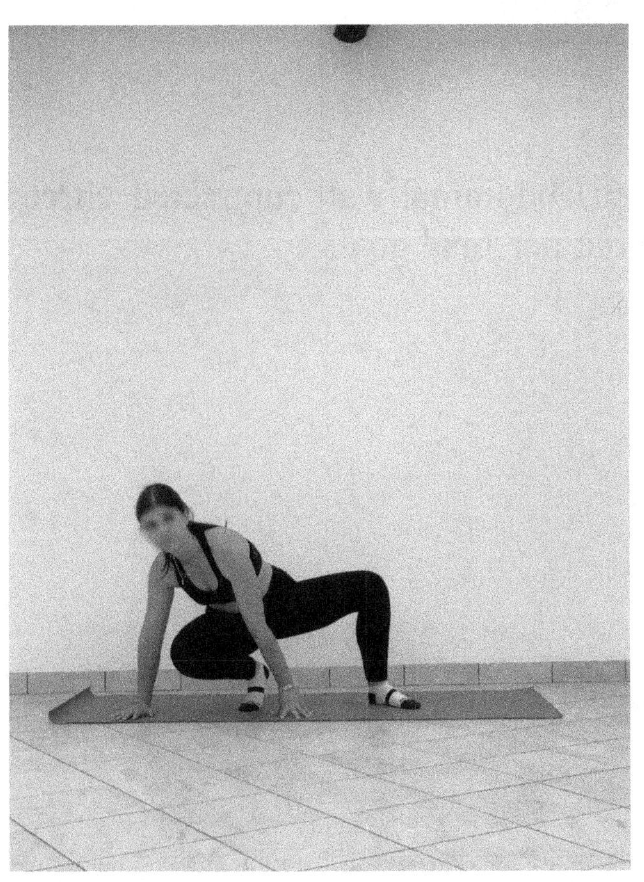

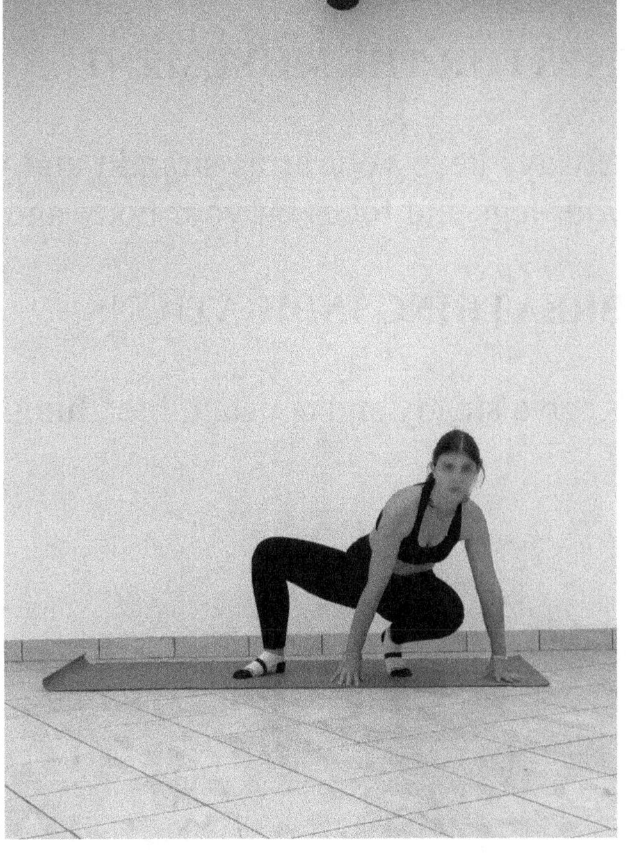

30 - DYNAMIC PLANK

BENEFITS:

- abdominal wall strengthening
- decrease in waist size

HOW TO PERFORM THE EXERCISE

1 Place yourself as you can see in the photo below

2 Bring the arms forward

3 Extend the legs and place yourself in plank position

4 Keep it for 3 seconds

5 Repeat the same movement from the beginning

TIPS FOR THE MOVEMENT

Always keep your arms straight and your abdominal wall contracted. Stretch your legs and focus on your body and your personal goals.

BREATHING INDICATIONS

Keep a steady and constant breathing.

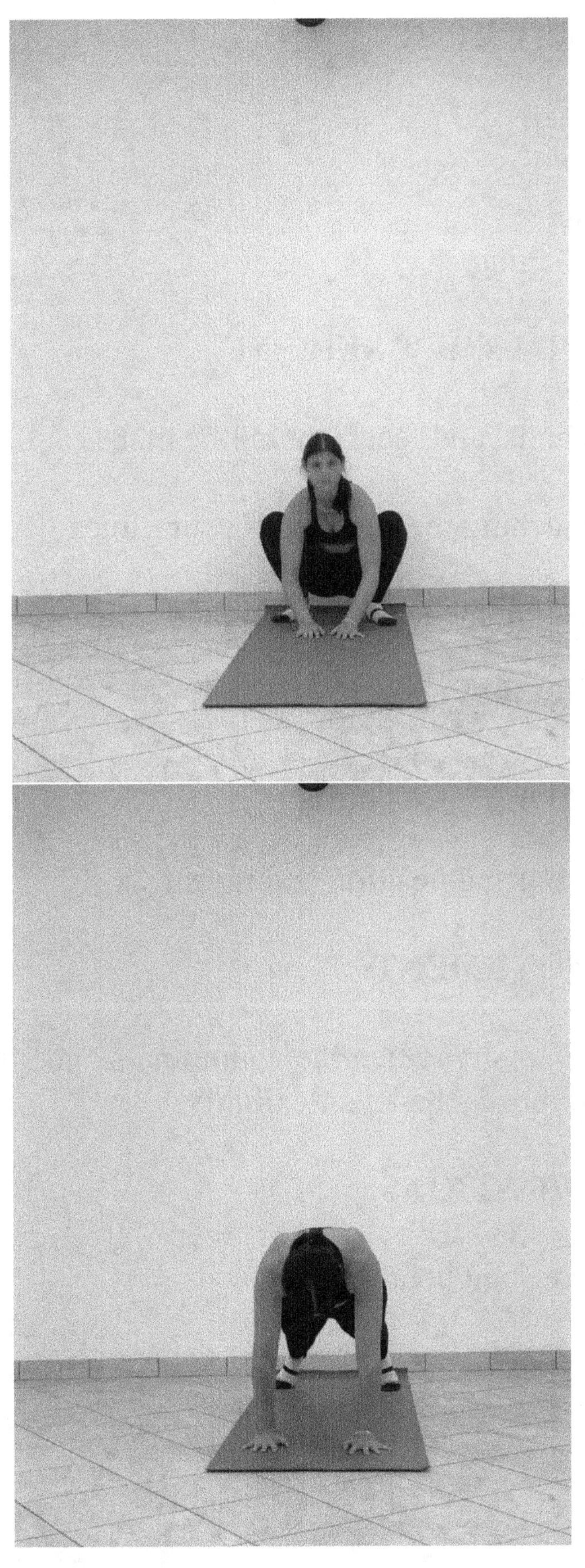

31 - STATIC STRETCHING

BENEFITS:

- back stretching
- triceps strengthening

HOW TO PERFORM THE EXERCISE

1 Place the knees, hands, and feet right on the mat

2 Spread the legs, touching the heels with your glutes

3 Bend forward, keeping the back well-straight

4 Rest the forearms on the mat

5 Keep this position for 5 seconds

6 Come back to the starting position and repeat

TIPS FOR THE MOVEMENT

This exercise goal is to strengthen the abdominals and stretch the muscles of the inner thighs to improve the legs flexibility.

BREATHING INDICATIONS

Keep a steady and constant breathing.

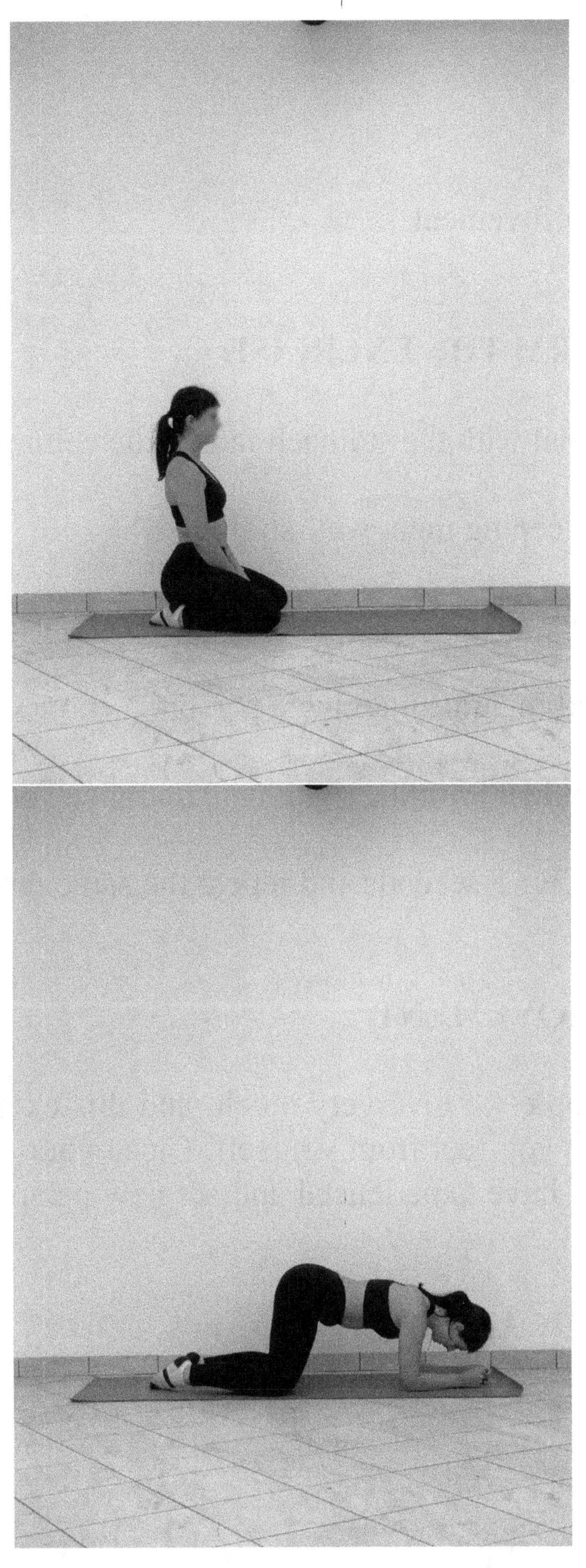

32 - HUG

BENEFITS:

- mind-body improvement
- spine relaxation

HOW TO PERFORM THE EXERCISE

1 Lie down on the mat with the stomach facing the ceiling

2 Spread the arms, keeping them well-straight

3 Face the palms upwards

4 Cross the arms and imagine hugging a person

5 Touch the left shoulder with the right hand and vice versa

6 Keep this position for 5 seconds and repeat the same movement from the beginning

TIPS FOR THE MOVEMENT

We usually hug people we love very much, and this exercise wants to make you feel all the love you feel from yourself. Close your eyes and think of all the good things you have experienced and set new personal and professional goals.

BREATHING INDICATIONS

Take deep breaths.

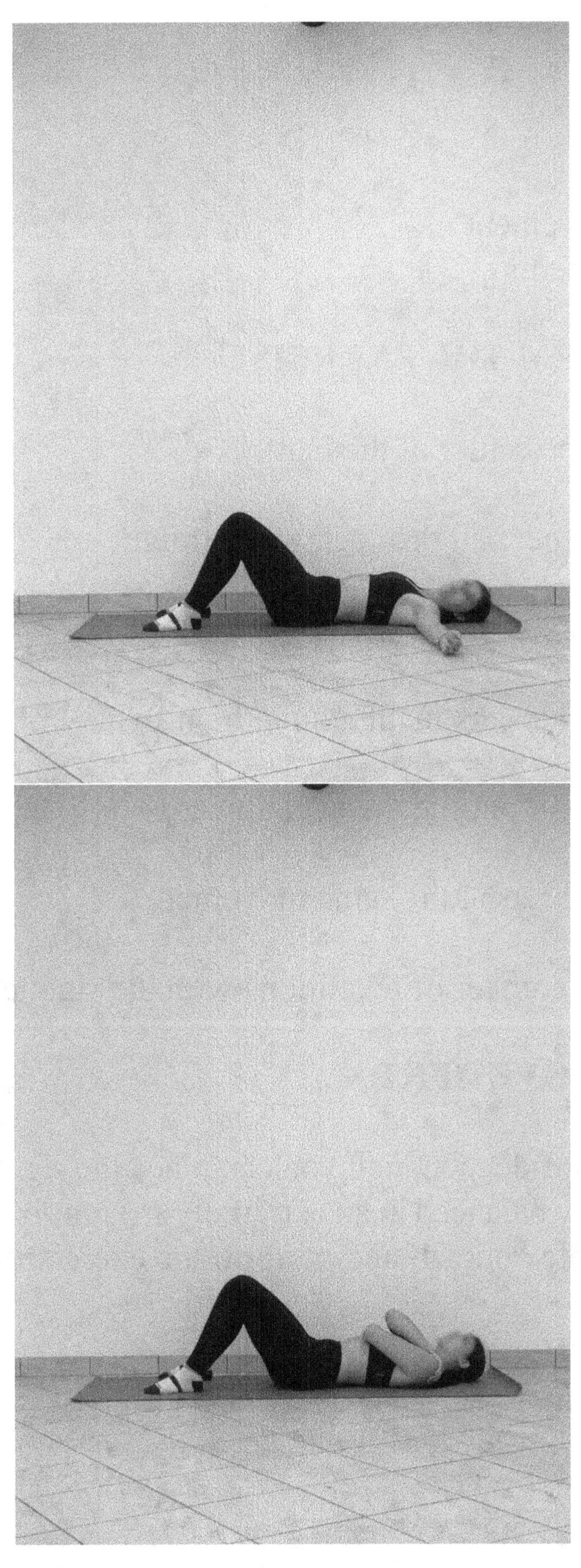

33 - CROSS

BENEFITS:

- balance improvement
- calves strengthening

HOW TO PERFORM THE EXERCISE

1 Place yourself at the center of the mat

2 Keep the feet together and the back well-straight

3 Raise the left knee, keeping it still

4 Raise the arms to the side, maintaining them tight

5 Contract the left calf, putting the heel upwards

6 Lower the foot and repeat the same movement

7 Conduct the same number of repetitions with the right calf

TIPS FOR THE MOVEMENT

If you do not feel confident enough you can place the right hand on the wall to have support and stay balanced in an extremely straightforward way. However, I suggest you evaluate yourself and perform the exercise without support.

BREATHING INDICATION

Keep a steady and controlled breathing.

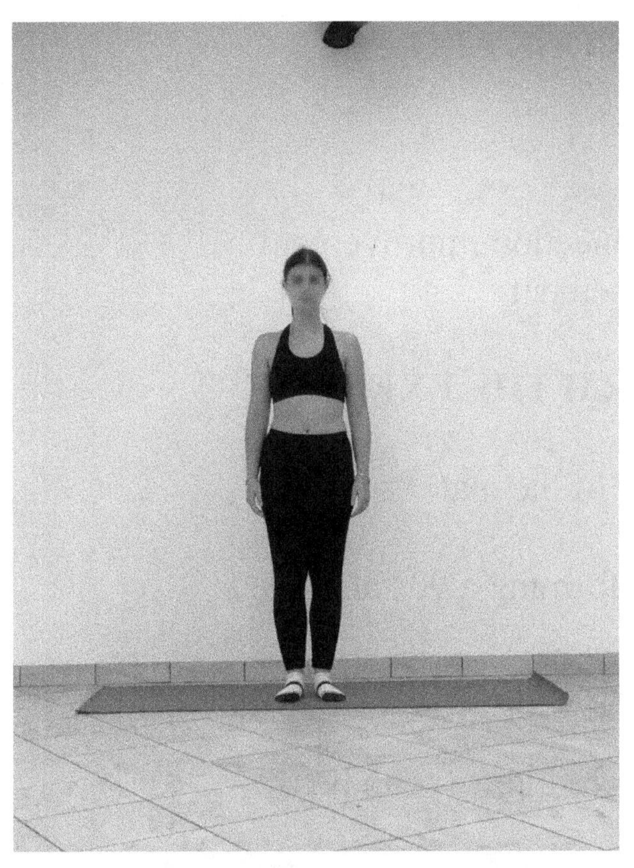

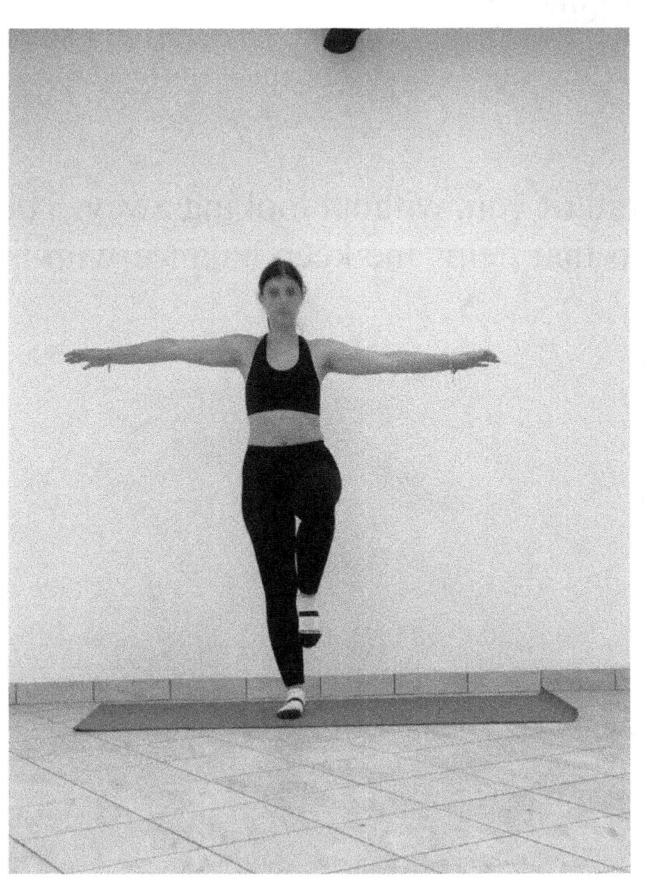

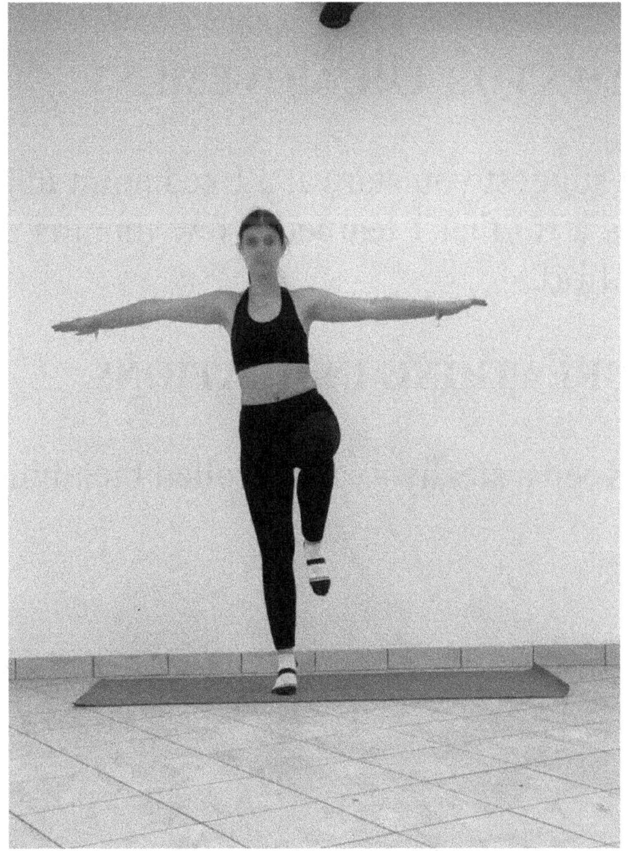

34 - BALANCE ON ONE LEG

BENEFITS

- mind-body connection improvement
- balance increasement

HOW TO PERFORM THE EXERCISE

1 Stand in the center of the mat

2 Raise the arms by forming a 90° angle

3 Slide the right foot down your left leg

4 Keep this position for a few seconds

5 Keep the arms well-straight, changing legs

TIPS FOR THE MOVEMENT

I suggest you stare at a fixed point in front of you, without looking away. This is a tip that I learned a few months ago that helps me keep balance with no effort.

BREATHING INDICATIONS

Keep a steady and controlled breathing.

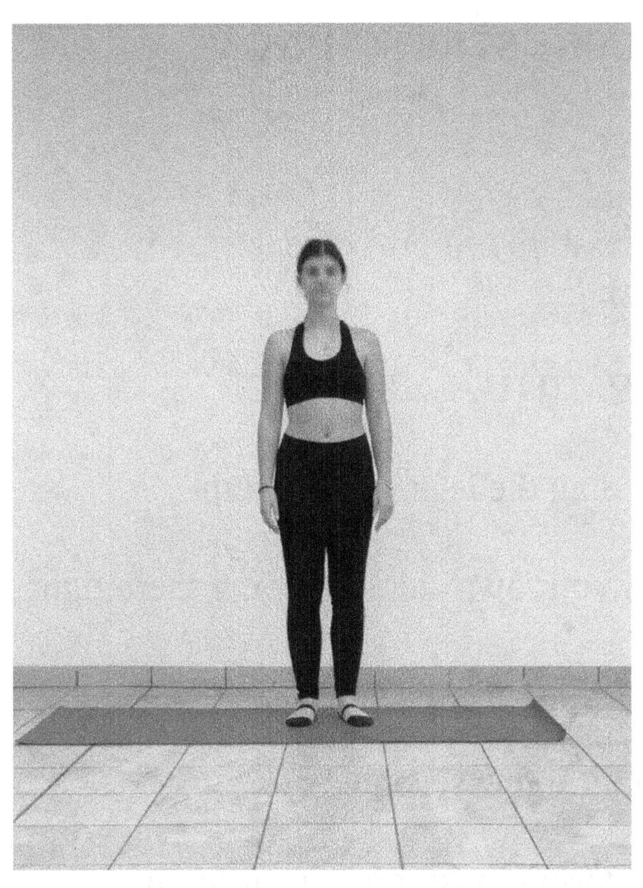

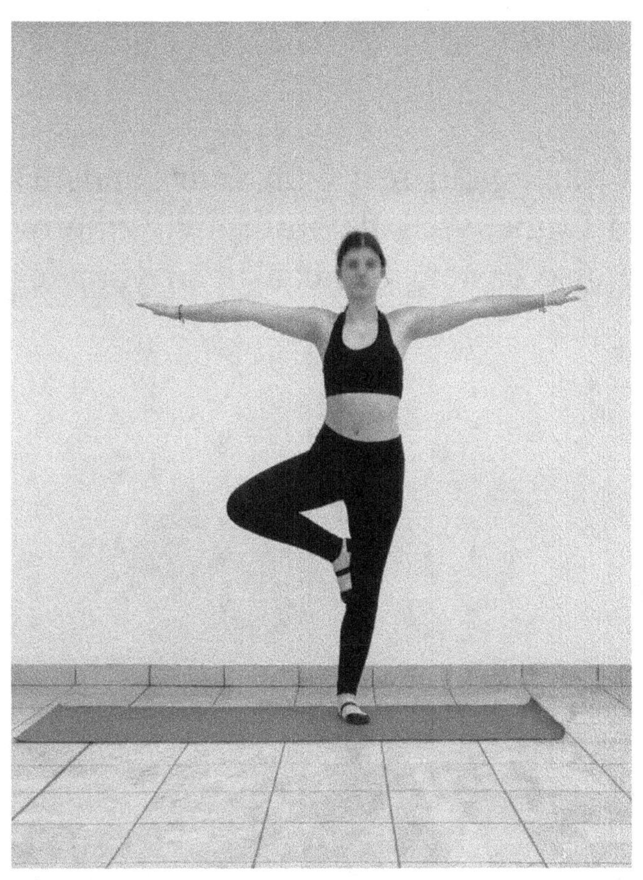

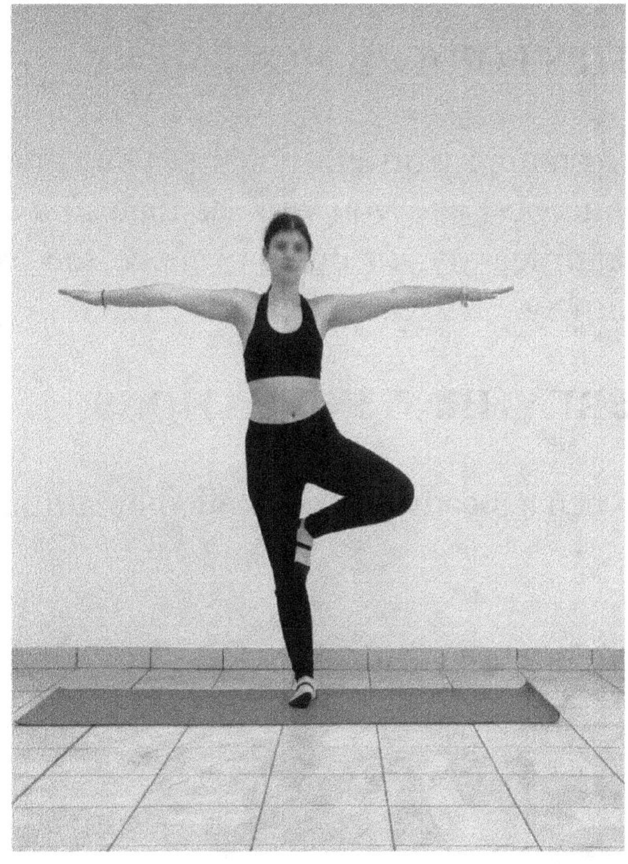

35 - COMPLETE LEGS STRETCHING

BENEFITS

- mobility and flexibility improvement
- femoral stretching

HOW TO PERFORM THE EXERCISE

1 Sit on the mat, keeping the legs well-straight

2 Extend the arms at your own sides, keeping them tight

3 Bend forward, touching the feet with your hands

4 Hold this position for a few seconds

5 Come back to the starting position, repeating the movement

TIPS FOR THE MOVEMENT

Do not be worried if at first you cannot touch your feet with your hands. Do your best and you will see that, in a short time, your flexibility will improve significantly. In order to make the exercise easier, you can bend your legs slowly.

BREATHING INDICATIONS

Keep a steady and controlled breathing.

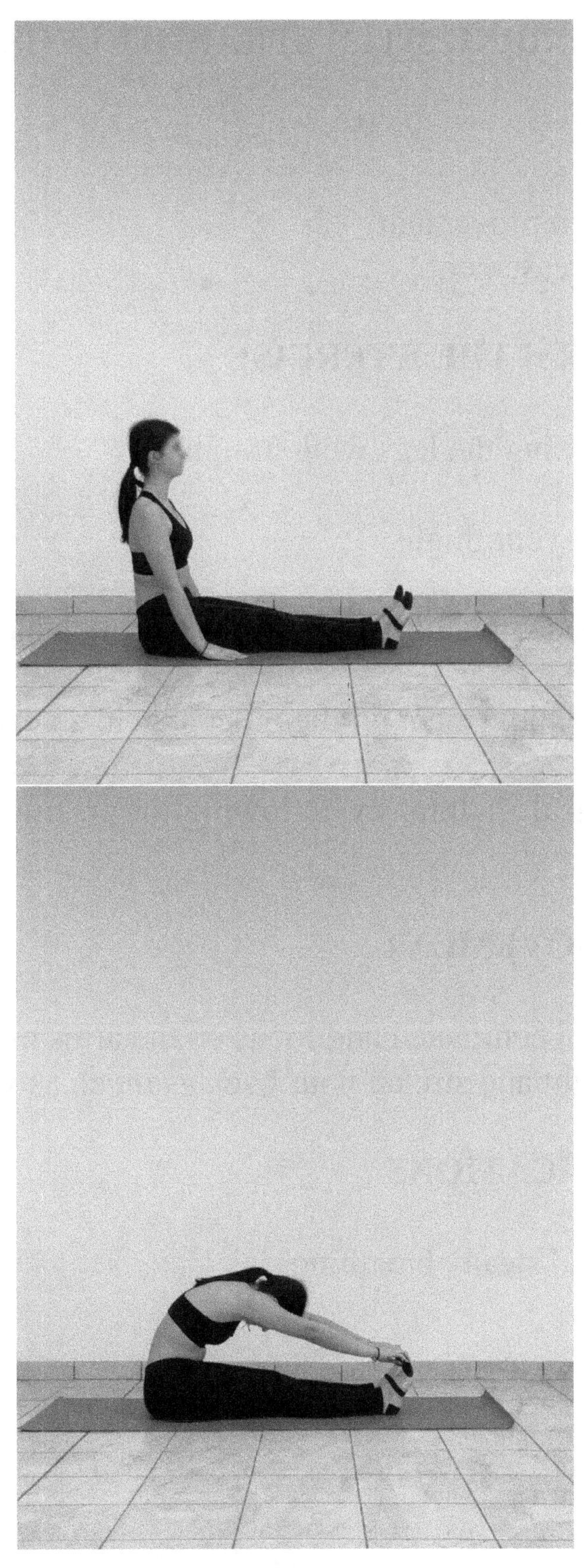

36 - LATERAL BENDING WITH STRAIGHT LEGS

BENEFITS

- joint mobility improvement
- abdominal increasement

HOW TO PERFORM THE EXERCISE

1 Sit on the mat, keeping the legs well-straight

2 Place the hands on your thighs

3 Bend to the right side, touching the floor with both hands

4 Carry out the same movement on the other side in a very dynamic way

5 Find your own ideal rhythm, by following the instructions present in this program

TIPS FOR THE MOVEMENT

Keep your abdominal contracted and focus on the arms movement, by holding your legs well-straight and stretch your back as much as you can.

BREATHING INDICATIONS

Keep a controlled and steady breathing.

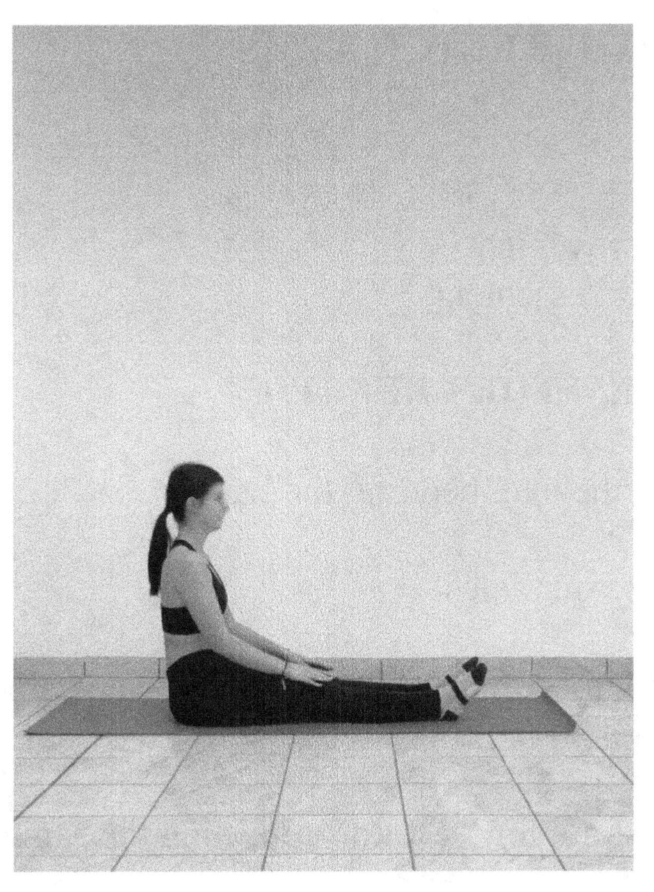

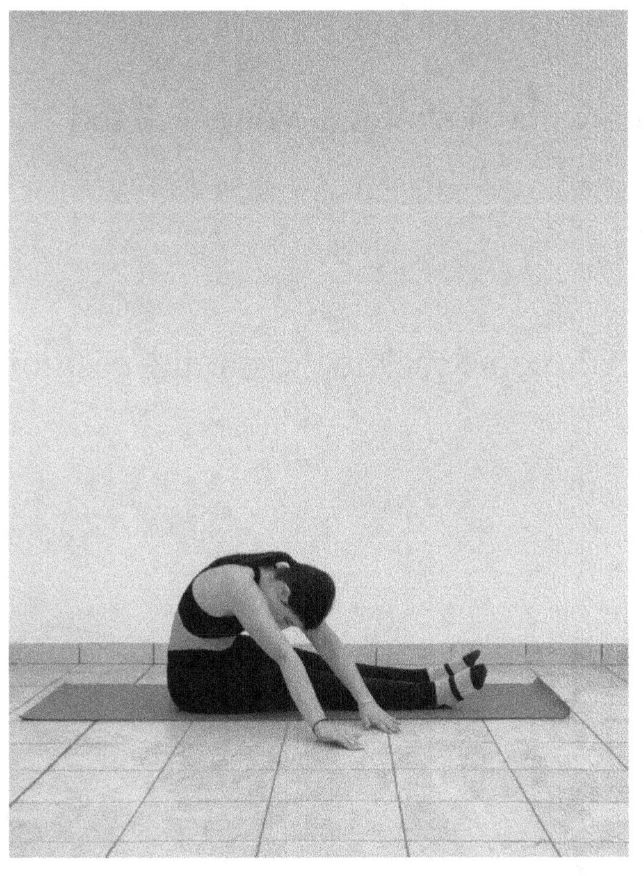

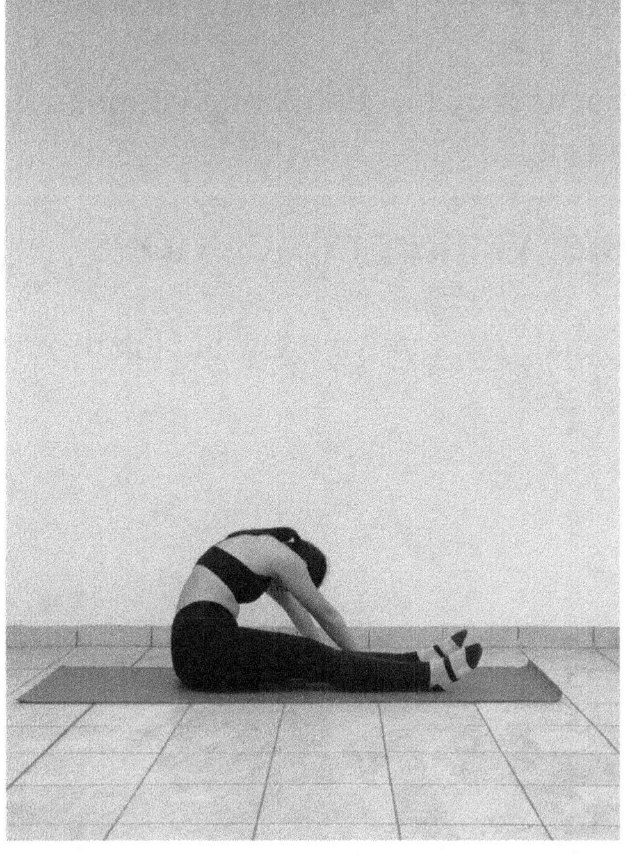

37 - CRUNCH WITH STRETCH ARMS

BENEFITS

- abdominal improvement
- coordination increasement

HOW TO PERFORM THE EXERCISE

1 Rest your back on the mat, bending the legs

2 Extend the arms at your sides

3 Carry out a crunch, touching the knees with the hands while you are keeping the arms well-straight

4 Hold this position for a few seconds, repeating the same movement

TIPS FOR THE MOVEMENT

Focus only on contracting your abdomen without straining your neck too much.

BREATHING INDICATIONS

Exhale once you crunch and inhale once you come back to the starting position.

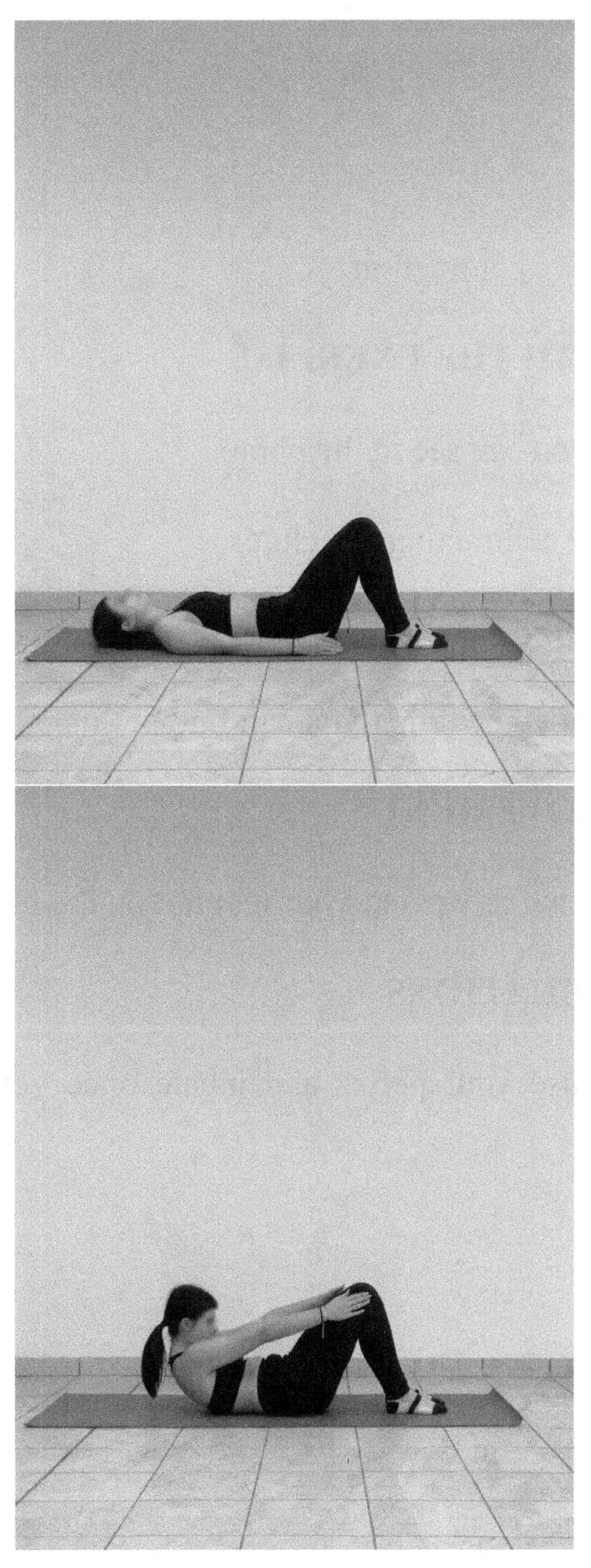

38 - BRIDGE

BENEFITS

-   glutes toning
-   quadriceps active contraction

HOW TO PERFORM THE EXERCISE

1 Place yourself as you can see in the photo

2 Raise the pelvis by contracting the glutes

3 Hold this position for a few seconds

4 Repeat the same movement that you can find in this program

TIPS FOR THE MOVEMENT

Keep your palms facing down and your feet flat on the mat.

BREATHING INDICATIONS

Exhale once you raise your pelvis and inhale once you come back to the starting position.

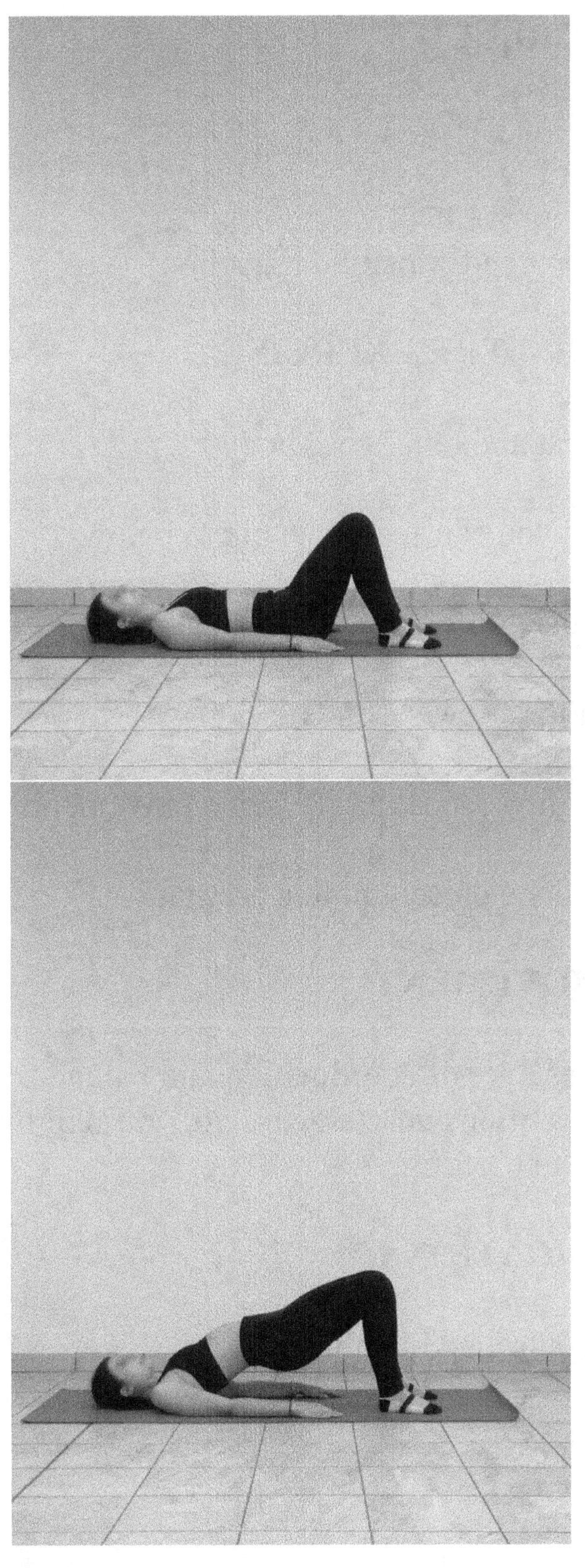

39 - COMPLETE CRUNCH

BENEFITS

- coordination improvement
- abdominal toning and waistline reduction

HOW TO PERFORM THE EXERCISE

1 Lie down on the mat and relax your body

2 Stretch the arms as you can see in the photo below

3 Bend the knees, raising the arms at the same time

4 Hold this position for a few seconds

5 Find your own rhythm, repeating the same movement

6 Follow the instructions present in this program

TIPS FOR THE MOVEMENT

This exercise requires a lot of coordination and balance; in fact, I suggest you carry out the first repetitions very slowly. So, you will understand exactly the movement you need to perform.

BREATHING INDICATIONS

Keep a steady and controlled breathing.

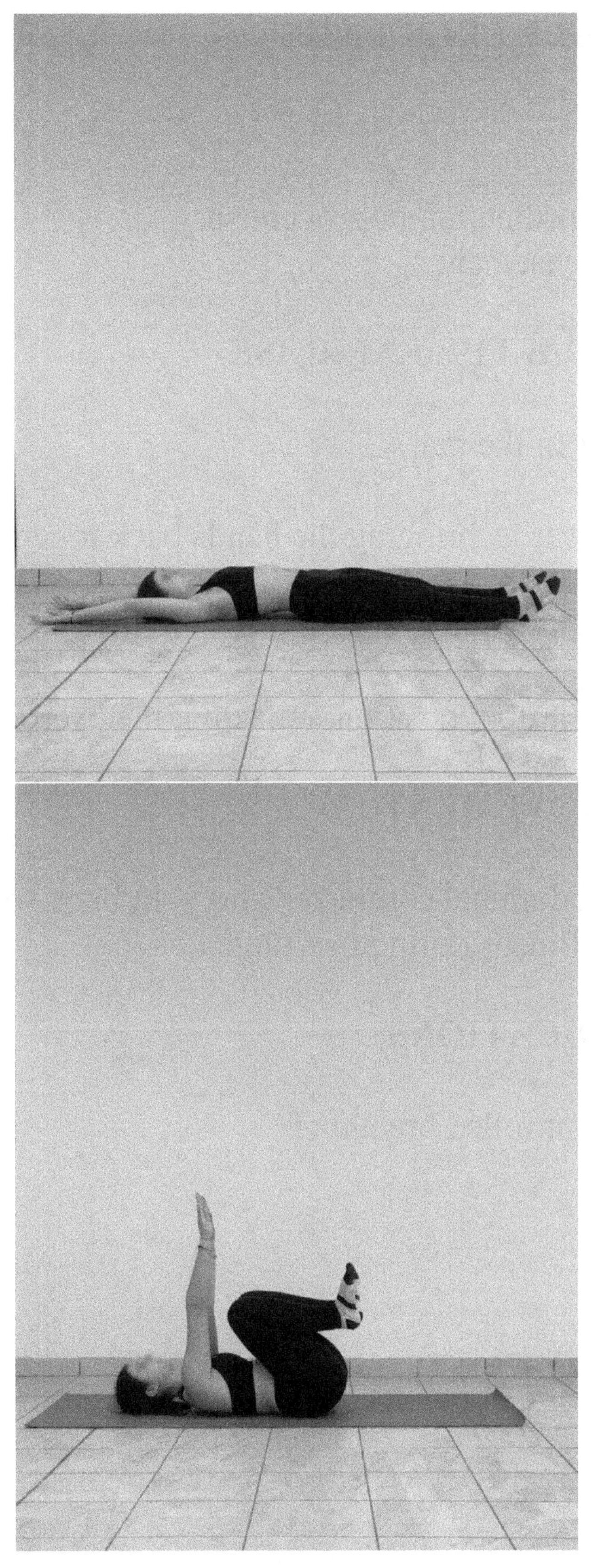

40 – STATIC SINGLE LEG LUNGE

BENEFITS

- balance and coordination improvement
- stabilizers increasement

HOW TO PERFORM THE EXERCISE

1 Stand in the center of the mat

2 Raise the arms upwards, bringing the hands back together

3 Bend the legs, touching the mat with the right knee

4 Come back to the starting position, repeating the exercise with the other leg

TIPS FOR THE MOVEMENT

Always keep your abdominal contracted and your back well-straight. Contract your glutes and quadriceps during the lunges.

BREATHING INDICATIONS

Keep a steady and controlled breathing.

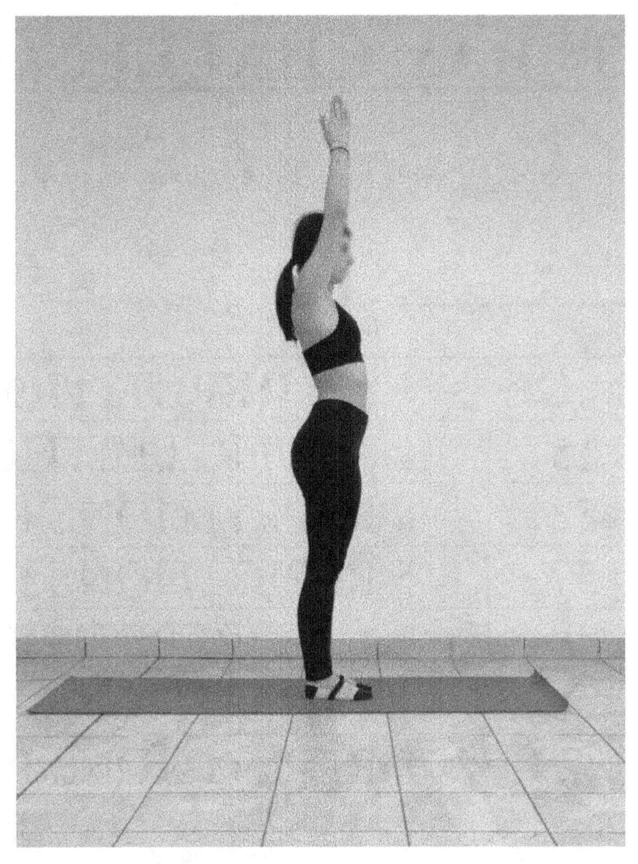

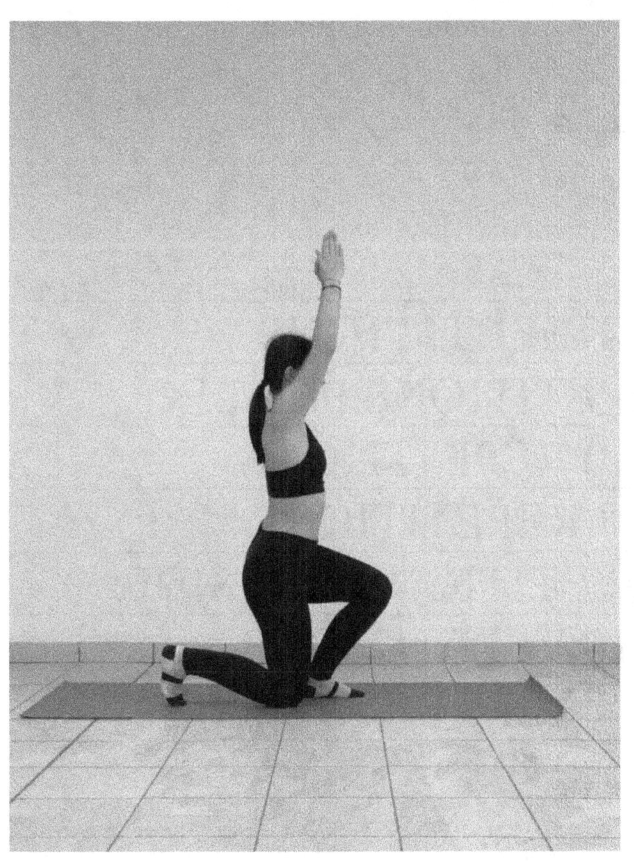

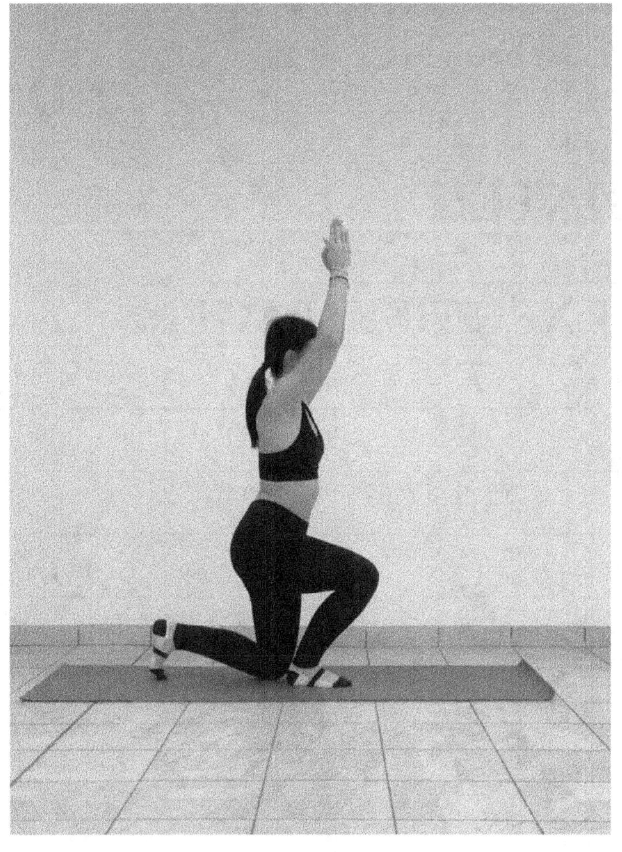

30 DAY CHALLENGE

DAY 1

DATE: _______________

EXERCISE	PAGE	REPETITIONS	V
8	15	10 REPETITIONS	
27	53	8 REPETITIONS PER SIDE	
29	57	5 REPETITIONS PER SIDE	
5	9	12 REPETITIONS	
13	25	8 REPETITIONS PER LEG	
4	7	8 REPETITIONS PER SIDE	

DAY 2

DATE: _______________

EXERCISE	PAGE	REPETITIONS	V
7	13	8 REPETITIONS PER LEG	
35	69	10 REPETITIONS	
30	59	8 REPETITIONS	
1	1	10 REPETITIONS PER SIDE	
18	35	10 REPETITIONS	
22	43	8 REPETITIONS	

DAY 3

DATE: ___________

EXERCISE	PAGE	REPETITIONS	V
34	67	10 REPETITIONS PER SIDE	
40	79	8 REPETITIONS PER LEG	
23	45	5 REPETITIONS PER SIDE	
7	13	8 REPETITIONSPER LEG	
5	9	12 REPETITIONS	
1	1	10 REPETITIONS PER SIDE	

DAY 4

DATE: ___________

EXERCISE	PAGE	REPETITIONS	V
15	29	3 REPETITIONS	
32	63	15 REPETITIONS	
23	45	5 REPETITIONS PER SIDE	
8	15	10 REPETITIONS	
6	11	8 REPETITIONS PER LEG	
2	3	12 REPETITIONS	

DAY 5

DATE: _______________

EXERCISE	PAGE	REPETITIONS	V
16	31	8 REPETITIONS PER LEG	
38	75	8 REPETITIONS	
25	49	5 REPETITIONS	
11	21	8 REPETITIONS	
9	17	15 REPETITIONS	
3	5	10 REPETITIONS	

DAY 6

DATE: _______________

EXERCISE	PAGE	REPETITIONS	V
17	33	3 REPETITIONS	
39	77	8 REPETITIONS	
26	51	20 REPETITIONS PER LEG	
12	23	8 REPETITIONS PER SIDE	
10	19	8 REPETITIONS PER SIDE	
4	7	8 REPETITIONS PER SIDE	

DAY 7

DATE: _______________

EXERCISE	PAGE	REPETITIONS	V
19	37	10 REPETITIONS	
35	69	10 REPETITIONS	
27	53	8 REPETITIONS PER SIDE	
18	35	10 REPETITIONS	
14	27	8 REPETITIONS PER SIDE	
13	25	8 REPETITIONS PER LEG	

DAY 8

DATE: _______________

EXERCISE	PAGE	REPETITIONS	V
21	41	10 REPETITIONS	
24	47	8 REPETITIONS	
39	77	8 REPETITIONS	
36	71	8 REPETITIONS PER SIDE	
28	55	8 REPETITIONS	
20	39	5 REPETITIONS PER SIDE	

DAY 9

DATE: _____________

EXERCISE	PAGE	REPETITIONS	V
33	65	8 REPETITIONS PER LEG	
30	59	8 REPETITIONS	
40	79	8 REPETITIONS PER LEG	
37	73	8 REPETITIONS	
29	57	5 REPETITIONS PER SIDE	
22	43	8 REPETITIONS	

DAY 10

DATE: _____________

EXERCISE	PAGE	REPETITIONS	V
39	77	8 REPETITIONS	
21	41	10 REPETITIONS	
24	47	8 REPETITIONS	
15	29	3 REPETITIONS	
38	75	8 REPETITIONS	
31	61	10 REPETITIONS	

DAY 11

DATE: _______________

EXERCISE	PAGE	REPETITIONS	V
15	29	3 REPETITIONS	
36	71	8 REPETITIONS PER SIDE	
1	1	10 REPETITIONS PER SIDE	
33	65	8 REPETITIONS PER LEG	
30	59	8 REPETITIONS	
22	43	8 REPETITIONS	

DAY 12

DATE: _______________

EXERCISE	PAGE	REPETITIONS	V
37	73	8 REPETITIONS	
32	63	15 REPETITIONS	
25	49	5 REPETITIONS	
19	37	10 REPETITIONS	
16	31	8 REPETITIONS PER LEG	
11	21	8 REPETITIONS	

DAY 13

DATE: _______________

EXERCISE	PAGE	REPETITIONS	V
40	79	8 REPETITIONS PER LEG	
19	37	10 REPETITIONS	
35	69	10 REPETITIONS	
27	53	8 REPETITIONS PER SIDE	
18	35	10 REPETITIONS	
13	25	8 REPETITIONS PER LEG	

DAY 14

DATE: _______________

EXERCISE	PAGE	REPETITIONS	V
21	41	10 REPETITIONS	
24	47	8 REPETITIONS	
38	75	8 REPETITIONS	
36	71	8 REPETITIONS PER SIDE	
28	55	8 REPETITIONS	
20	39	5 REPETITIONS PER SIDE	

DAY 15

DATE: _______________

EXERCISE	PAGE	REPETITIONS	V
33	65	8 REPETITIONS PER LEG	
30	59	8 REPETITIONS	
2	3	12 REPETITIONS	
37	73	8 REPETITIONS	
29	57	5 REPETITIONS PER SIDE	
22	43	8 REPETITIONS	

DAY 16

DATE: _______________

EXERCISE	PAGE	REPETITIONS	V
39	77	8 REPETITIONS	
21	41	10 REPETITIONS	
24	47	8 REPETITIONS	
16	31	8 REPETITIONS PER LEG	
5	9	12 REPETITIONS	
31	61	10 REPETITIONS	

DAY 17

DATE: ________________

EXERCISE	PAGE	REPETITIONS	V
1	1	10 REPETITIONS PER SIDE	
36	71	8 REPETITIONS PER SIDE	
8	15	10 REPETITIONS	
33	65	8 REPETITIONS PER LEG	
30	59	8 REPETITIONS	
22	43	8 REPETITIONS	

DAY 18

DATE: ________________

EXERCISE	PAGE	REPETITIONS	V
12	23	8 REPETITIONS PER SIDE	
32	63	15 REPETITIONS	
25	49	5 REPETITIONS	
19	37	10 REPETITIONS	
16	31	8 REPETITIONS PER LEG	
11	21	8 REPETITIONS	

DAY 19

DATE: _______________

EXERCISE	PAGE	REPETITIONS	V
30	59	8 REPETITIONS	
19	37	10 REPETITIONS	
35	69	10 REPETITIONS	
27	53	8 REPETITIONS PER SIDE	
18	35	10 REPETITIONS	
13	25	8 REPETITIONS PER LEG	

DAY 20

DATE: _______________

EXERCISE	PAGE	REPETITIONS	V
21	41	10 REPETITIONS	
24	47	8 REPETITIONS	
3	5	10 REPETITIONS	
36	71	8 REPETITIONS PER SIDE	
28	55	8 REPETITIONS	
20	39	5 REPETITIONS PER SIDE	

DAY 21

DATE: _______________

EXERCISE	PAGE	REPETITIONS	V
33	65	8 REPETITIONS PER LEG	
30	59	8 REPETITIONS	
9	17	15 REPETITIONS	
37	73	8 REPETITIONS	
29	57	5 REPETITIONS PER SIDE	
22	43	8 REPETITIONS	

DAY 22

DATE: _______________

EXERCISE	PAGE	REPETITIONS	V
39	77	8 REPETITIONS	
21	41	10 REPETITIONS	
24	47	8 REPETITIONS	
16	31	8 REPETITIONS PER LEG	
12	23	8 REPETITIONS PER SIDE	
31	61	10 REPETITIONS	

DAY 23

DATE: _______________

EXERCISE	PAGE	REPETITIONS	V
8	15	10 REPETITIONS	
36	71	8 REPETITIONS PER SIDE	
5	9	12 REPETITIONS	
33	65	8 REPETITIONS PER LEG	
30	59	8 REPETITIONS	
22	43	8 REPETITIONS	

DAY 24

DATE: _______________

EXERCISE	PAGE	REPETITIONS	V
15	29	3 REPETITIONS	
32	63	15 REPETITIONS	
25	49	5 REPETITIONS	
19	37	10 REPETITIONS	
16	31	8 REPETITIONS PER LEG	
11	21	8 REPETITIONS	

DAY 25

DATE: _________________

EXERCISE	PAGE	REPETITIONS	V
6	11	8 REPETITIONS PER LEG	
19	37	10 REPETITIONS	
35	69	10 REPETITIONS	
27	53	8 REPETITIONS PER SIDE	
18	35	10 REPETITIONS	
13	25	8 REPETITIONS PER LEG	

DAY 26

DATE: _________________

EXERCISE	PAGE	REPETITIONS	V
15	29	3 REPETITIONS	
24	47	8 REPETITIONS	
1	1	10 REPETITIONS PER SIDE	
36	71	8 REPETITIONS PER SIDE	
28	55	8 REPETITIONS	
20	39	5 REPETITIONS PER SIDE	

DAY 27

DATE: ________________

EXERCISE	PAGE	REPETITIONS	V
33	65	8 REPETITIONS PER LEG	
30	59	8 REPETITIONS	
4	7	8 REPETITIONS PER SIDE	
37	73	8 REPETITIONS	
29	57	5 REPETITIONS PER SIDE	
22	43	8 REPETITIONS	

DAY 28

DATE: ________________

EXERCISE	PAGE	REPETITIONS	V
24	47	8 REPETITIONS	
39	77	8 REPETITIONS	
38	75	8 REPETITIONS	
21	41	10 REPETITIONS	
9	17	15 REPETITIONS	
31	61	10 REPETITIONS	

DAY 29

DATE: _______________

EXERCISE	PAGE	REPETITIONS	V
10	19	8 REPETITIONS PER SIDE	
33	65	8 REPETITIONS PER LEG	
30	59	8 REPETITIONS	
22	43	8 REPETITIONS	
15	29	3 REPETITIONS	
36	71	8 REPETITIONS PER LEG	

DAY 30

DATE: _______________

EXERCISE	PAGE	REPETITIONS	V
8	15	10 REPETITIONS	
25	49	5 REPETITIONS	
19	37	10 REPETITIONS	
11	21	8 REPETITIONS	
16	31	8 REPETITIONS PER LEG	
24	47	8 REPETITIONS	

TRACKING CHART

DAY	DURATION OF THE WORKOUT	MOTIVATION (HIGH/LOW)	ARE YOU PROUD OF YOURSELF ?
DAY 1			
DAY 2			
DAY 3			
DAY 4			
DAY 5			
DAY 6			
DAY 7			
DAY 8			
DAY 9			
DAY 10			
DAY 11			
DAY 12			
DAY 13			
DAY 14			
DAY 15			

DAY 16			
DAY 17			
DAY 18			
DAY 19			
DAY 20			
DAY 21			
DAY 22			
DAY 23			
DAY 24			
DAY 25			
DAY 26			
DAY 27			
DAY 28			
DAY 29			
DAY 30